Bedtime Sto[ries for] Adults

Soothing Sleep Stories with Guided Meditation. Let Go of Stress and Relax. Mrs Robinson and other stories!

Sleep Academy

Mrs Robinson!

It would be a normal Friday afternoon, you'd be in your house probably playing video games or jerking off to porn, and you'd look outside your window and see me, your hot older next-door neighbour having trouble with her lawnmower. You would get the ingenious idea in your mind that if you helped me, maybe you could live out all your fantasies about me. You would hurry outside and check in on me, asking me what was wrong and if you could help in any way, I would tell you that my lawnmower was broke and I had to have this done by the time my husband and all his friends got here, or he would kill me. You, of course, would happily tell me that you had no problem in getting your own lawnmower over here and doing it for me, and I would be so grateful for you and say that I would pay you if you did it. You would quickly get to work cause you'd think the more time you spent joking around, the less of a chance, we would have to do something together, you would go and get your lawnmower and then come back over and get to work. I would watch you from inside, admiring your body and how good you looked without a shirt on, you would quickly now the lawn and hope that I would invite you in after like in all those porno's you watched it happen. You would finish up, and fix yourself before you knocked on my door and told me you had finished with it and that you were gonna head back home and clean up but I would invite you in, of course, so you could have some lemonade, and I could pay you. So we would walk back to my kitchen, and I would hand you a glass, and I would grab my purse and ask you how much you wanted, and you wouldn't hear me because you were too busy staring at my tits through my small tank top and my ass in the short-shorts I was wearing that didn't cover all of my ass. I would snap at you and ask how much you wanted and you'd make your move, saying you didn't want any kind of money and I would ask what kind of payment you wanted, and you'd say something more along the lines of sexual payment. I would have to think about it for a second, I mean you are underage and if my husband ever found out he would be so angry, then again your cock might be better than his, and you might be able to please me, unlike my husband. I would agree to it, and I would come around the counter and get really close to you, pressing my lips to yours as I reached down and rubbed my hand over your already hard cock. I would grab your cock through your shorts and pull you back to my room, I would push you down on my bed and tell you to stay still, and I would crawl on top of you and rub my hand over your cock through your pants very slowly before I pulled them down and ran my lips over the outline of your cock through your boxers very slowly, looking up at you as I did it and your cock would twitch a little and then I would pull your boxers down. I would start by rubbing myself against you with my shorts still on, and you'd love that feeling of my clothes against your bare cock I would keep grinding myself against you, and you would enjoy every second of it, feeling my pussy against yours through my shorts it would make your cock throb. I would then move off of you and just take your cock in my hand, wrapping my hand around your shaft really tight, my nails digging into the skin and you'd wince at it, whimpering a little cause you're not used to anything but the feeling of your own hand around it. I would start jerking you off really slow, my other hand on your balls squeezing them I would spit on it too, making it extremely sloppy and the spit would get everywhere, and you'd be enjoying yourself very much, watching me your hot older neighbour doing something you'd only been able to dream about and then I would start jerking you off faster being extremely rough with you, pulling and tugging on your cock and showing your balls no mercy when I squeezed them. I would jerk you off for a little longer before I had to stop so you wouldn't cum then and there. I would give it a little break before I continued again, your cock would still be hard when I crawled on top of you and whispered in your ear that there was something special I wanted to do and you'd have to be extremely open-minded for both of us to enjoy it. I know you'd agree to anything I wanted, I'm sure you'd enjoy all of this anyways you're a sick little boy. I would tie your hands up to the headboards along with your legs so I could have good access to your cock and balls. I would start my kissing at your chest and being really slowly as I made my way down all the way to your

4

cock and I would kiss along your cock and suck on your balls a little boy before I leaned back and balled my fist up, looking you straight in the eyes as I brought my fist down against your balls and you'd let out a loud groan, pulling at your ties because you wanted to protect yourself, but I would tell you to stop squirming so much if you didn't want to hurt your wrists and then I would do it again, and you would notice that you were actually enjoying this a lot. I would keep looking at you as I did it and then I would start being nice again, rubbing my hand over your cock and balls really slowly before I hit them again, I would spit on your cock and tell you how it's not much better than my husbands, and that's not a compliment. I would then stand up and rub my foot over your balls slowly before I stepped down on them a little, watching you closely to make sure you wanted it. Of course, you would; you loved everything I was doing to you. I would then continue to step on them, not putting too much pressure on them cause I wanna start you out small. After I did that for a little while I would pull my shorts off and sit back down and pull my panties aside and rub myself against you, trying to make myself feel good a little bit. I would then ask if you wanted me to fuck you and you'd say yes, and I would ride you, being extremely rough about it. I would slam myself down against you every time I went down, and I would grind my pussy against your with your cock inside me, and you would love my tight pussy; you would go out of your mind because it feels so amazing. I would let out a few fake moans, your little cock is not very satisfying, and I would have to fake it to keep your little boy feel safe. I would keep on fucking you, rubbing myself against you and slamming myself down my ass moving against your balls as I did. You would tell me that you're close to coming and I would quickly get off you and start jerking you off again, my hand wrapped tight around your shaft, being very rough tugging and pulling on it very hard and then you'd cum all over yourself, and I would untie you and let you clean yourself up because my husband would be here soon and you needed to get back home, but if you come back another day we might be able to do it again. I would make you swear not to tell anybody not even your little gamer buddies and you wouldn't if you wanted to keep this fantasy up. You would hurry home and probably dream about this day for the rest of your little boy life.

Dom School Girl

We see each other around school all the time, and we only ever interact with each other when it has to do with me putting you in your place which is quite

Often nowadays. It would be like any other day just going to class minding my own business, and you would be doing the same up until like 5th period when you decided to make some stupid remark on something that was very important to me, and it would send me over the edge. I would wait until it was time for lunch and I would grab you after you left the classroom by your tie and it would tighten around your neck, and you'd choke a little bit and take you to one of the empty classrooms again, and you'd be confused about course you hardly ever know what's going on. I would push you up against the door, and I would ask you why you said what you did earlier, why you would make that kind of a joke on something so serious. You would be confused at first before you remembered what you said and I would look you in the eye and shove my knee between your legs, tilting my head s little bit as a asked again, why would you say that kind of thing? And you'd just stutter out some bullshit apology like you didn't know how wrong it was of you to say that kind of thing. I would tell you that I wanted you to hurt yourself instead of me doing it for you, I would push my knee up into your balls, and I would look at you and nod a little, and you would push yourself down against my knee really hard and keep on doing that until it hurt and make your cock sore. You would ask me to stop because this was embarrassing how I was making you do this and I would just tell you to keep on going, and harder this time. You would keep on doing it, and I would reach down and grab your cock in my hand, tugging on it as you pushed yourself down onto my knee, groaning every time you did, and I would tell you to do it harder, I know you can do better than that little boy. You would slam your balls down against my knee probably so hard you'd beg me to stop again, and I would tell you no that we aren't done until I said so. I want you to hurt I want you to learn from this because you make far too many stupid remarks in class and I am growing very tired of it. So I want you to feel this pain and remember every time you even think about saying something. I want you to get a filter on that mouth of yours. I would push your shoulders down so you would go down harder, you're a baby about it. I want you to shed a couple of years cause it hurts so bad, I want you to be a man and take it. I would keep on pushing you down, and every time your balls hit my hard knee, you would let out a little whimper like a puppy crying for its mommy. I would jerk your cock off a little bit, and I would grow tired of your lack of ability to hurt yourself so I would start doing it myself, I would shove my knee up into your balls, and you'd double over, and I would just push you back up so you could take another hit. Your cock would grow really sore, and it would be hurt, probably turning red. I would keep on going though; I want the pain to be so bad it feels good, so good you cum in your pants. I would push my knee farther up and with more force than I ever had, I would let out a little grunt when it hit your balls, and you'd cry out and probably cry a little. I would keep going, though until I felt your cock throbbing. I would say that you have a little baby cock and u know you are craving this, I know how much you're into this you dirty little boy. You would tell me how bad you needed to cum, and you would beg me to let you, but I would refuse. You do not deserve to cum; I want you to keep this cum for a couple of days until I come back and finally let you release. I would then tell you to start doing it again, forcing yourself down on my knee as I jerked you off really fast and you would tell me it was getting to be too much that if you went any longed you would cum right there so I would take a step back and look you in the eyes and tell you to never ever say that kinda stuff again or this punishment would feel like a walk in the park. I would then lean up and slap you across the face and tell you goodbye until next time and kiss your lips and leave the room.

Mrs Robinson and Dom School Girl!

It would be a Friday afternoon, and I would come to pick you up after school since your parents were away for the weekend and you needed a ride home. I would pull up to the school and wait outside my car, my arms folded over my chest, waiting for you to get out. You would walk out the building, and I would see you with another little girl with her skirt up way too high trying to pull off the cute school girl look, and she would be all over you, and then I would see her drag you off somewhere, and I would follow behind the two of you at a distance watching as she touched all over you and I would get a little bit jealous. I would watch as she pulled you into a room and I would watch as she pushed you up against the wall and tried to dominate you, her weak little arms trying to keep you against the arm and she would be sloppy with how she touched you and soon it would become too much so I would burst in the room and I would just go off. I would tell the little bitch to get out of the room and never talk to you again, I would slap her across the face and that she should go home and fix herself. Then I would handle you, you unfaithful little boy who thought he could get away with sneaking around with a little bitch; I'm much smarter than you don't you know that? I would make you sit down in one of the empty chairs, and I would grab a ruler off the desk and slap it against my hand and then I would look at you. I would ask you what you were doing, and you wouldn't know what to say, you would just sit there with that dumb look on your face, and it would take everything in me not to slap it off you. I would sit down on the teacher's table and cross my legs, cocking an eyebrow at you and I would ask again, what were you doing with her. You would try your best to get the words out that it just happened, that one day she just threw herself on you and you didn't know how to stop her and she would give you a lot of attention and would dominate you as I do. So I would just nod my head a little and look at the ground before I stood back up and walked over to the desk and leaned over, giving you a clear view down my shirt and I would place the ruler under your chin and push your head up to look me in the eyes, and I would speak very softly and slowly when I told you that after I'm done with you, you'll never even look at another girl. I would stand back up and grab you by your tie and yank you out of your seat, the tie tightening around your neck and I would drag you over to the corner and throw you down, and I would tell you to strip out of

11

your clothes, everything but your tie and boxers. You would quickly do what you were told, very afraid of what I was gonna do to you. After you stopped down I would make you stand back up and lay against the table, and you'd do it, and I would rub the ruler down your chest slowly, slapping it against your body as I went down and when I got to your cock I would run it across it slowly, and when I got to your balls, I would smack the end against it. I'd keep a careful eye on you as I did, slapping the ruler against your balls repeatedly, making you count each time I did it. I would then grab your tie and pull you up a little bit, looking you in the eyes and I would ask how many times you and she had done things, and you would tell me about four, so I am gonna bring you so close to cumming you wanna cry four times. I would tighten the tie around your neck and shove it in your mouth and push you back down against the table and tell you to shut up. I'd start off first just by touching on your cock, slowly rubbing my hand across it, squeezing your balls a little bit and jerking it off some, I would be very slow, taking my time as I made you really hard for me, I wanted to drag this one out really long. I would lean down and spit on your cock, jerking it off with my hand really tight around it, my nails digging in as I leaned down and sucked on your balls, biting on them a little bit and then I would jerk you off a little bit faster, squeezing your balls really tight as I did, slapping them a couple of times. You'd tell me that you wanted to cum and I would just jerk you off faster, and I would tell you that you're not coming at all today. You'd be begging me to let you cum, and I would just shake my head, jerking you off until the very last second, and then I would punch you right in your balls, and you'd groan out and have to hold in your cum. I would wait a little bit before I started touching you again because I wanted this to last a long time. I would grab you by your tie and pull you down off the table, and I would push you down on the ground, using my foot to make you lay down, I would pull your boxers off the rest of the way, and I would tell you that this is how a real woman takes control of her man. I would press my heel into your stomach, watching your face as you groaned out in pain. I would drag it down your cock slowly, pressing the tip of my heel into it. I would take a step back before I rubbed my foot over your balls slowly, watching you closely before I smashed all my weight down against your balls and you'd sit up a little bit, trying to cover yourself but I would push you back down and tell you to stay still, or you're not gonna like it. I would repeat the process, rubbing my foot over your balls before I pressed all of my weight on them. You would be in so much pain you'd be on the verge of tears, but I wasn't gonna stop, you need to see what a real woman can do for you. After a while the pain would turn into immense pleasure, and you would start enjoying the feeling of it, your cock would start twitching, and I would keep doing it over and over again, occasionally rubbing my heel along your shaft and you would come so close to cumming you'd be yelling out my name begging for it, and I would shake my head again, continuing to step on your balls until I had to stop so you wouldn't cum. I would pick you back up and press you against the wall, shoving my knee between your thighs, your balls just above it and I would look you in the eye and tell you that I wanted you to do some of the work now, and you would beg me not to make you do it, I know how much doing this embarrasses you, and that's why I love it so much. I would tell you that you do this or I'm leaving and you would never get me again. So, of course, you would pick doing it, you would slam yourself down against my knee, you balls being smushed as you did it, and you would start off small, and I would just keep on making you do it again and again until I thought it was hard enough. You would keep building it up, and I would just keep telling you to go harder because I know you can do better than that baby. You would keep smashing yourself down against me, moaning out my name every time you did it. I would whisper in your ear how angry I am with you and I'm not sure if even this will be good enough to make up for what you've done, cheating on me with a dumb school girl. After I said that you would start slamming yourself down harder, finally as hard as I wanted and you'd be in so much pain, your cock would become so sore and your balls almost numb from the pain. I would call you a dirty boy a bad boy and I was gonna punish you some more for what you've done to me. Im not very pleased with how you've been acting and I would reach down and grab your cock, digging my nails in and I would jerk you off until you were hardly able to breathe because of how bad you wanted to cum and as soon as your cock started twitching I would let go and back away from you, and you would slump down against the wall a little because all of this would make you tired. I would then tell you to get back into the table and wait for me there. I would watch as you crawled back on and I would walk over to you, undoing your tie and I would use it to tie your hand to the leg of the table, slipping out of my underwear and using them for your other arm. I'd warn you that if you stretched out my nice undies, you wouldn't be very happy about it. So I would then crawl on top of you, rubbing myself against your cock slowly, dragging my sharp nails along your chest as I ground my pussy against your cock slowly. I would slam myself down against you, my ass smacking against your balls and I would tell you that I was gonna do this until you were so close you shed tears. You would get so frustrated, being so close to my pussy but not being able to be inside of me, I would rub myself against you and make myself feel good for once, using your cock. I would keep slamming myself down against you, pressing my ass against your balls and I would finally make myself cum. I would keep pressing myself against you before I got off and grabbed your cock, jerking you off really fast, my nails digging in and scraping along your shaft as I jerked you off and I would punch your balls as I did it and you'd tell me you needed to cum, and I'd tell you that you needed to shut up. I would bring you so close you shed a tear because of how much pain you were feeling

15

but also the odd pleasure of it all. So right when you were about to cum I would stop grab my panties and head towards the door, looking back and telling you that I'd be out waiting in the car and it would be in your best benefit to get out there soon. You'd have to untie your tie and get dressed quickly, or I would leave you at school, and you'd have to walk home, and as soon as we got back, I would be teaching you another lesson at your house.

Dinner with Mrs Robinson.

Friday night at a dinner party that your parents invited my husband and me too. I would dress really nicely, probably in something a little provocative, fitting into my milf next-door neighbour status, putting on some heels to finish it. You would probably be watching me, then again I did leave my blinds open for a reason. My husband and I would arrive a little early; he hates being late; it's part of his whole personality, douche bag husband that treats me like crap. We would bring a nice bottle of wine, in hopes to impress your parents that even though we are younger, we still have "style", his idea again. You would come downstairs and look so handsome; I would watch you carefully and smile a little because you had no idea what was in store for you tonight. You would be jealous as you saw my husbands arm wrapped around your waist, wishing that it was you that could do that, but you were kept in private. We would all sit down in the living room as we waited for dinner to finish, you would have to watch as my husband touched on me and talked about our many adventures and you would only grow more jealous, wishing again that you could experience this kind of things with me, this anger will be good for later. We would have a couple of glasses of wine, not you just the adults, and then we would make our way into the dining room where I would be seated right across from you. We would talk about many things, places we vacation and stuff we both have done, and you'd just sit quietly and watch. Luckily my legs are long enough to reach under the table and reach your crotch; I would rub my foot against your cock and balls slowly, still keeping my conversation up with your parents, my husband leaning against me, trying to give off the idea that we were actually a happy couple. I would keep rubbing my heel against you, occasionally pushing it against your balls and you would have to keep the straightest face you could or else you would give us away. I would get you really hard for me just by doing that, pressing my heel into your balls, being really rough with them and I would rub your cock a little bit until your cock was throbbing and in a little bit of pain. I would go into the kitchen to get something to drink, and you'd follow me, a dumb move on your part, but I will let it pass. I would push you up against your counted my knee pressed close to your balls, and I would tell you that I'd come back for you, later tonight I wanted to see you again. I would quickly grab your cock through your pants and squeeze it before turning back around and making my way to the table again. The adults would keep talking, my husband would probably end up having a little bit too much to drink as usual, and I would have to excuse us and take him

18

home. I would give you a little look, the one where I'm telling you that I will be back for you later and stay up for me. You'd watch as I carried my drunken husband across your lawn and back into my house. Your jealousy would make you very angry, and your parents would wonder what you were so upset about, and you'd just brush them off and go back to your room, in hopes you could see me through my window as I undressed. I would bring my husband inside, throw him down on our bed and let him pass out for the night, knowing he wouldn't be up until tomorrow for work. I would get undressed, looking across into your room and I would rub my tits a little, flashing a small smile when I saw you watching in awe. I would mouth the word, "later." and you would stay up and wait for me to come back to you. I would go and change into something else; you would watch of course as I had to lay down in bed with my drunk husband and wait a few hours until I could bring you back to my house. A few hours would pass, and it would be around 12, and I would come back to my window, try to get your attention so you would sneak out and come to my house. As soon as you made it past your parents snoozing in the living room and to my back door, I would let you in and press you up against my wall, pressing my lips to yours and we would make out for a good while before I reached my hand down and grabbed your cock, squeezing it really tight as I jerked you off. I would keep your cock in my hand as I led you to my living room, pushing you down onto the couch, I would crawl on top of you and rub myself against you slowly, kissing you to keep you quiet in case my husband decided to get up. I would rub my pussy against your hard little cock, until you were throbbing for me again. I would ask you how it was for you at dinner, and you'd tell me how jealous you got seeing my husband and me together and him being all touchy with me, and I would tell you to shut up, you know what you were getting into. I would push my knee in between your legs and rest it on top of your balls gently, and I would look you in the eyes and ask how you liked me touching you, and you'd say that you loved it, as usual, and I would nod a little bit before I said that I was gonna do it some more. I would press my weight down into your balls, and you'd let out a little groan, the one that I love so much. I would rub my hand along your cock as I kept pressing my weight down against your balls more and more and you would enjoy every second of it, and you might get a little bit too loud so I would have to cover your mouth, so we don't get caught. After a while of teasing you and torturing your balls, I would probably give you a little break, so I would lean down and suck on your cock a little bit, looking up at you as I did and you would just lay back and enjoy every second my mouth is wrapped around your little cock, bobbing my head and my eyes not breaking contact with yours. I would move my head down even more and take in all of your cock, gagging a little bit on it before I lifted my head back up. Then we would hear footsteps moving around, and I would tell you to be quiet, and I would turn the tv on and throw a blanket on top of you as my husband came downstairs, and I would ask him what he was doing, and he would say he was getting a drink and then before he left he would come to give me a kiss goodnight right after I sucked your cock. He would go back upstairs and probably pass out again. I would pull you out from under the blankets and flash a little smile before I would take your cock in my hand, wrapping it around it tightly my nails digging in as I jerked you off really hard and I would use my free hand to squeeze your balls really tight, and I'd lean down and whisper in your ear how dirty you are and how much I love what a naughty boy you are for me. I love how much you enjoy being hurt, and how vulnerable you are, I love taking control of you. I would sit up a little bit and push your boxers back up so I could turn around and rub my ass against your balls really slowly, I might even let you pull your cock out a little and rub it against me. You would tell me that you wanted to cum soon and I would say no, I wanted to make this last longer. I would slam myself down against you, rubbing myself against you really slowly. I would then turn back around and tell you that I wanted you to do some of the work, that I wanted you to press your balls against my knee until you came for me. I would lay back a little, keeping my knee up so you could rub your balls against it. You would be really slow and gentle to yourself at first, barely doing anything to your little cock and balls. I would tell you to do it again, and harder this time. I want you to make it hurt so bad. You would try and slam yourself down harder on me, and I would say to go harder that you can do better than that, I know you can be a big boy. You would start to slam yourself down really hard on my knee, letting out these little whimpers every time because it hurt so bad and I would tell you to keep going that I know you love how it's feeling. You would do it over and over again until your cock became really sore and I would tell you to go until you came for me. You would slam yourself down on my knee until you were in tears, almost begging me to let you release. I would tell you to go for it, and you would cum all over the place, on yourself on my leg probably getting s little bit on my couch. You would be so tired from it that you would ask to stay over and I would tell you maybe another time when my husband is not home. I would have to clean you up before you left to go back home, and the stain on the couch would not be coming out. I would walk you to my back door and tell you that I had a nice time and I would kiss you goodbye. You would walk back home, and I would go up to my room and watch as you got into your room and as you looked across at me before you got into your bed, and then so would I, both of us waiting for the next time that we got to see each other, hoping that it would be soon.

The Hot Principal

My Monday morning would start out normal, faxes paperwork and making the rounds around the school. It would be completely average until I came across some spray painting of the words "the principal has nice tits" and I would hurry back to my office so I could look over the security tapes and see who did that. You would be pulled out of class and taken to the office and wait for me to call you in. I would wait a little bit before I opened my door and invited you in, closing the door behind you and I would ask you to take a seat. You would sit down, and I would walk around my desk, turning my computer monitor around to show you what was on it, and I would hit the play button. You would watch the clip showing you spray painting the wall with what you did and then after you watched it I would turn it about around and I would sit on the edge of my desk. I'd ask you why you did that and if you really thought you'd get away with that and you would just tell me that you thought I had great tits and was hoping that if you did it I would bring you in and you could stare at them longer. I would cross my arms over my chest and shake my head, looking you dead and the eye and I would tell you that you could get suspended from school for doing this, that you wouldn't be able to return until next year for destruction of property. You would just shrug your shoulders and roll your eyes, and that would be it for me. I would stand up and grab your face and look you in the eyes, and I would tell you that when I was finished when you, you'd be admiring a lot more than just my tits. I would push the things on my desk aside and push you down against it, locking the door, and I would stand at the edge of my desk, looking down at you as I ran my fingers across your torso, lifting your shirt up a little bit, my actions would be slow and soft so you would be very unsuspecting to what I would do next. I would keep running my hand along your body, being extremely slowly until I made it down to your cock where I would rub my hand over it slowly before I slammed my fist down against it and you would groan and ask me what I was doing, and I'd ask whether you'd rather do this or be suspended cause the choice was up to you, I just figured you'd rather do this. That would shut you up quickly; I would put a pen in your

mouth for you to bite down on so you'd be quiet, I would keep doing it, over and over again every time my fist hit your balls it would be even harder than the last. I would pull your pants down along with your boxers, running my nail along your shaft slowly before I dug them into it, squeezing your cock really tight in my hand and I would jerk you off really quick, you would just bite down on that pen really hard, trying your best to keep all the noises in, I mean we don't want anybody hearing you now do we? I would use my free hand to grab your balls, pulling and tugging on them as I continued to jerk you off. I would then crawl on top of you, undoing my shirt a little so my tits would spill out, and I would rest my knee right in between your legs, pushing it up closer to your balls, and I would ask you if seeing my tits now were worth what you did to school property, and you would stick by your answer and tell me that you wanted me to see it so I would know and find you. I would then press my knee down on your balls and dig my nails even further into your cock, continuing to press my weight into your balls and then take it off and then press it back in again and every time I leaned off of them I would ask you again, and I would do this until you finally said the right answer. You would tell me how sorry you were for doing that to my school and that it would never ever happen again and I'd tell you that if it ever did, I would do this again. I would then smash my knee against your balls, jerking your cock off really fast, pulling on it and you'd tell me that you needed to I'm, and I would tell you no, you can't cum yet. I would sit up a little, taking one of my feet and pressing it against your balls, putting all my weight on them as I spit on your cock, I would dig the pointy edge of my heel into it, and you would beg me to stop, your little balls wouldn't know how to handle this because you've never gotten this kind of attention before and I would tell you that you can only cum after your balls ache so bad they go numb. I would keep pressing my foot into your balls, pressing my hand on your cock and I would feel it throbbing, and you would tell me that you were going numb and that it hurt so bad, but I know you we're secretly enjoying it, you're a sick little kid that loves when a woman older than him takes control. I would continue jerking you off, stepping into your balls and when I felt like it was time I would let you cum, and you'd cum all over yourself. I would get off and tell you to clean up and go back to class, and if you ever did that again, you'd know what would happen.

Sadistic Step Mommy

You would be coming home from school, probably stressed from all the work your teachers were giving you before the break that was coming up. I would be sitting in the living room, watching tv as you walked in the door and you'd let out a big sigh, slamming your books down on the kitchen table, and I would be startled. I would quickly walk over to you, resting my hand on your shoulder as I asked you what was wrong and if I could help any. You would tell me that it was just all the homework you had to do, it was stressing you out, and I would sit down next to you and rub my hand over your arm, and I would offer to help you. You'd shrug me off and tell me that you didn't need any help from me, that you'd get along just fine. I would lean back and cross my arms, shaking my head a little bit, and I would look at you and ask if that's any way to treat your stepmother. You would roll your eyes and tell me that I was hardly a mother to you at all since I'm closer to your age than your fathers. I would correct you and tell you that I'm actually closer to your dads, that 36 wasn't that young. You'd laugh it off and stand up and gather your things, and I would grab your arm and pull you back into your seat and tell you that you aren't allowed to treat me like this, that I'm an adult and you should treat me with respect. You'd tell me that you wouldn't do anything of the sort and that would be it for me, I would stand up and push your things off the table, and I'd say that after I am done with you, you would have nothing but respect for me. You would look at me very confused, and I would tell you to get up and sit on the table, and you would shake your head, trying to get up and leave, but I would grab your arm and dig my nails in, looking you straight in the eye and I would repeat myself, get on the table. This time you would listen to me, climbing up on the table and I would part your legs and get in between them, I would grab your chin and make you look up at me, and I would say, "You're gonna learn your place little boy, and I'm not gonna stop until I say so and if you interrupt me I will get even angrier." You probably wouldn't know what to do so you would just nod your head, and I would smile a little bit, reaching my hand down to rub you through your pants and you would kinda push me off, asking me what I was doing and I would tell you I'm doing what I wanted, and you need to sit still so I can. I would keep rubbing you through your pants, squeezing your cock a little bit through them and you would get hard for me really fast because truthfully you're very into it. You'd had fantasies about your hot stepmom; ever since your dad introduced us, you've wanted something like this to happen. I would undo your button and zip down the zipper, pulling your pants down a little along with your

28

boxers and I would pull your cock out, taking it in my hand, squeezing it really tight my long nails digging into your skin. You would let out a little noise, and I would just laugh if you think this hurts. I don't know if you'll be able to handle what I want to do. I would continue to jerk you off really fast, tugging and pulling at your cock, using my free hand to squeeze at your balls really tight. I would pull your pants down all the way and push you a little, so you would lay back, moving your boxers back up, so your cock was inside them again. I would crawl on top of you, sitting on your lap and I would start grinding myself against you, rubbing my pussy against your cock really hard, my ass would push against your balls, and I would bounce a little bit, smashing myself against you until I could feel your cock throbbing through the fabric. I move off of you a little bit, my legs in between yours and I would pull your boxers all the way down, rubbing my hand against your cock slowly, and I would tell you that you're gonna have to trust me, cause what I'm gonna do is probably gonna hurt a lot at first, but you've gotta relax. I would put my knee over your balls gently, leaning down so I could spit on your cock and I would slowly press my weight into your balls, and you'd let out a groan, sitting up a little bit, but I would push you back, telling you to stay still. I would jerk your cock off as I slowly pressed my weight into your balls, putting more pressure onto them each time I did. It would hurt you at first, making you wanna cry a little bit but you would grow to enjoy the pain, craving it even. I would then press all my weight into your balls, jerking your cock off really fast, digging my nails into it as I did. I would then start smashing my knee into your balls, and you would groan out in pain but also a pleasure. I would then tell you that I had something I wanted you to do for me. I would make you get up and come to the couch, and I would sit down, and I would have you sit down on one of my legs, I'd tell you that I wanted you to smash your balls against my leg, and you'd be probably against it at first, not wanting to humiliate yourself in front of me, a little worried I would go off and tell all my friends about my pathetic little stepson. I'd reassure you to trust me, that I wanted you to do this for your step mommy. You would just nod and start bouncing yourself against my leg, I would tell you to grab your cock and jerk yourself off, and then I'd say, "Come on can't you do better than that? This is pathetic, you're a baby about this." and then you would start doing it harder, smashing your balls against my leg so much it hurt, jerking your cock off as you did it. I would just sit back and watch you, unbuttoning my blouse and touching my tits a little bit as you did. You'd tell me that your cock was twitching and your balls were starting to go numb and I would just tell you to keep on going, no stopping until I said so. You would continue to do as you were told, smashing your balls against me, I would reach up and push on your shoulders so you would go harder, and you'd tell me you wanted to cum and I would say no, not yet you won't. I'd make you get up and go stand by the wall, and I would come towards you, I'd tell you to spread your legs and hold your cock-up. I would then swing my leg back and next thing you knew my foot was kicking your balls, you'd double over, and I'd tell you to stand back up and be a man. I would continue doing this until you were on the verge of tears. You'd tell me that your cock was aching and if you didn't cum soon you might explode. I would tell you to lay down on the floor and to jerk yourself off. I would stand above you, rubbing my foot against your balls slowly. I would then press all my weight into them, you'd let out a little noise, and I'd tell you to jerk yourself off until you come on yourself. I would keep stomping my foot down on your balls, pressing my foot into them extremely hard. It wouldn't take long for you to cum after that, and after you did, I would step off of them and tell you to get up and clean your filthy self off. I was done using you, and you will have gotten newfound respect for your step mommy. I would tell you to go back to your room and think about this, and I would probably go off to my own and call up one of my friends. You wouldn't be able to ever get this off your mind, always thinking about your stepmom busting your balls, hoping that the next time it happened would be soon.

Sadistic Step Mommy pt. 2

If you had gotten into trouble one day at school and were sent to the principal's office and I had to come to pick you up from school because you had to take some days off I would probably get pretty pissed off because it disrupted my day and also because you had gotten in trouble. Once I picked you up, I would ask you what you did, and all I would get was you ruined school property. I would grip the steering wheel with one hand; the other would be griping your cock so hard your face would scrunch up in pain, trying to hold in my anger until we got home. We would pull into the driveway, and I would get out and wait for you to come inside, I would lean up against the counter and look at you, tapping my foot against the floor. You'd give me one of those infamous "what?" looks and that would be it for me. I would grab you by your arm and pull you into your room, pushing you down on to the ground, straight on your ass and I would go off. Basically, telling you how much a disappointment this is how disappointed I am in your for doing this kind of thing, and what for? attention? you just got kicked out of school, and now you're going to miss things in class and fall behind. I would tell you to get your pathetic ass up and to lay on the bed. You would be a little scared, you'd never seen me this way, and you knew what happened the last time you upset me a little bit, but you would do as you are told. You would get up and lay down on the bed, and I would walk towards the edge of the bed, pulling your pants down really fast and then I would rip your boxers off and pull your cock out, wrapping my hand around it extra tight, my long nails digging into your skin, leaving little marks in their wake. I would jerk you off really fast, squeezing your balls extra tight and I would lean down and suck on your balls, looking up at you before I bit down on them, you'd groan out and try to push me off, but I would just bite harder before I stood bad up and crawled on top of you, pressing my knee into your balls harshly, putting all of my weight into it immediately, I would be so pissed I wouldn't care about easing you into things this time. I would grab one of your belts and tie your hands up to the headboard, shoving my underwear in your mouth so you'd be quiet. I would then slap around your cock around, punching your balls as well. I would take out all my anger that was build up from today on you sexually; I would squeeze your balls until my knuckles went white, I would scrape my teeth along your shaft really slowly not caring how bad it hurt you. I would keep reminding you how disappointed I was in you, how I knew you could do so much better than this and that I was doing this to teach you a lesson. I would then step up onto the bed a little, kicking my shoes off and I would step onto your balls, pressing the heel of my foot against them, bouncing my weight up and down on them, it would hurt you so bad, but you would also be really into it. I would then sit down on your cock, rubbing my ass against it, slamming myself down on you and then I would grind against you, you'd love the feeling of my dress pressing against your ass, that rough feeling against your cock would turn you on even more. I would then untie you, making you stand up so I could kick your balls a couple of times, managing to kick them harder enough you fell to your knees a couple of times. I would then I would push you up against the wall, your head hitting it and I would shove my knee right up into your balls. I would then tell you to jerk yourself off as I busted your balls, pushing my knee up into your balls and you'd double over, leaning on me and I would press you up against the wall again, telling you to stay fucking still, or I'll hurt you more. Your cock would get a little swollen from the abyss, and your balls would almost go numb from it. I would lean up and whisper in your ear how pathetic and disappointing of a son you are, how I could believe that I had to claim you sometimes. I would ask you again why you were punished, and you would finally tell me after about the third time of my kicking you square in the nuts. You'd tell me that it was saying something provocative and I would get even angrier, asking why the hell you would ever think that's a good idea. You would just shrug your shoulders and say that they had nice tits, so you wanted to let the world know. I would feel a little pang of jealousy so I would probably start kicking you in the balls again and you'd beg me to stop but I wouldn't until I felt like it. I would make you lay on the floor and start jerking yourself off, and I would watch until I finally would step on your balls and telling that you would cum this way for me and then you're grounded for a couple of days, you'd be spending lots and lots of time with me over the neck few days. We will have plenty of time for other lessons you need to learn. You'd tell me that you were close so I would step down even harder and then you'd cum all over yourself and then I'd leave the room, slamming it shut behind me. I would probably go check online to see what your principle looks like, curious as to who she was. You would just sit in your room, trying to decide if you loved that or not.

Bad Beach Boy

I would've just gotten to the beach, and already making its way into my shoes as I walked down the side of the beach. I would probably have my headphones in, I would have short shorts on showing off my amazing ass, and my bikini top would barely cover my tits. I would set my towel out and lay down on it, I would pull my tube of oil out, and I would start rubbing the oil on my body, hoping I would get a nice tan out of being here today. I would lay back, looking out at the beautiful ocean and I would mind my own business, just listening to music and tanning, enjoying my day when I would look over and notice you. You were just an average looking boy, seemingly normal until you looked a little closer, I would sit up a little to see if I saw correctly when I saw your hand in your swim trunks. I would look again, and sure enough, I was right, your hand was all the way in them, definitely jerking yourself off by the looks of it and I would get furious. Nobody can come to the beach without being looked at by a creep. I found you absolutely disgusting. I would stand up and walk over towards you, tapping my foot as I waited for you to notice me, I would clear my throat a little boy, and you would look up at me, your hand stopped moving in your pants immediately as you saw me and I would ask what you were doing, and you'd just tell me you were enjoying a day at the beach, the sun the sand the water. I would nod my head before I spoke again saying you were enjoying much more than just the beach, I would look down at your crotch, pointing at it and I would raise an eyebrow, and ask why you were jerking off in a public place in front of all these people, children even. You would tell me because it's a free country and you can do whatever you want when you want, and that would be it for me; I would grab you by your arm and start pulling you back towards my stuff, I would grab my things and pull you over behind some small sand dunes and tell you to sit down, I was gonna teach you a lesson on how to act in public since apparently your mother never taught you. I'd tell you that you were never gonna even think about touching yourself in public after I was done with you. You would be kinda scared, this woman you had just met was kind of threatening, and you'd wondered what you'd gotten yourself into. I would then get down on my knees and rub your cock through your pants, squeezing it a little bit before I pulled it out of your pants, jerking you off really fast and you would be a little shocked at what I was doing because I was mad a second ago. I would then tell you that what I was about to do would hurt, but your little pervert self would deserve every bit of it. I would then pull your pants down even further, wedging my knee between your thighs and I would rest my knee above your balls, and you'd ask what I was doing, and I would tell you to shut up, I would cover your mouth with my hand, and I would lean all of my weight into your balls, using my free hand to jerk you off. You would try and push me off a little, and I would give you a little looking telling you to stay down, and you would secretly like this, the fact I was in control. I would keep pressing my weight into your balls over and over again. I would whisper in your ear how much your tiny cock deserved to be treated like this, how much your pervy self deserved to feel this pain. It would just turn you on, even more, you would become so hard your cock started to throb, and your balls ached, I would keep jerking you off quickly, tugging and pulling on your cock, stomping my weight against your balls and you'd beg to come, but I don't want that yet, not at all. I would tell you to lay back on my towel, and I would get on top of you, grinding myself against you slowly at first before I slammed myself down against you, my ass slapping against your balls my pussy pressing down against your throbbing cock and you would beg to feel my right pussy around you, and I would say no, you're a creep, and you don't deserve my pussy, it's too good for this little cock. I would keep grinding myself on you, slamming my ass against your balls trying to force you closer to cumming than ever before in your life before I would take it all away from you. I would then move off of you and stand up a little bit, telling you to jerk yourself off while I did this. I would rub my foot against your balls, glancing down at you before I stepped down on them, all of my weight would be on your balls, and I would bounce on them a little bit, and you would be in so much pain, begging me to stop but also not wanting it at the same time. I would tell you to jerk yourself off harder; I saw how you did it earlier. I know you can do it better than that you little pathetic creep. I would keep on pressing my weight into your balls and then finally after you begged me half a dozen times to cum I would let you, all over your nice shirt.

I would then grab my things and remind you that it's a crime to do what you were doing in public and if you ever get caught again, the person wouldn't be as nice as me. I would then walk away, and you'd just sit there for a little bit, trying to figure out what the hell just happened and why on earth you liked it so much.

Cheater

In our small group of friends, it would be, me you and my best friend. You and my best friend were dating at the time, but the truth is you had always had a crush on me. Sometimes when we would all hang out when she would leave the room, you and I would get pretty handsy, but we would never do anything else, that is until one day when she had to go take care of something for a while, and she left us at her house, obviously not thinking much would happen, she was wrong. She would've just pulled out of the driveway, and we would be sitting on her couch in the living room. We would probably be watching Netflix, just chilling waiting for her to come back when you'd reach over and touch my leg, and I would look over at you and give you a look like no we can't do this. You would keep on trying, pulling me closer to you and you would whisper in my ear how much you've wanted this for so long and sometimes when you're with her, you come close to saying my name. After a while of you trying and failing, I would give up. I would pull your face closer to mine, and I would whisper that this could only happen one time before I would press my lips to yours, crawling in your lap. We would probably make out for a good ten minutes, and with me grinding against you, it wouldn't take long for you to get hard for me. I would continue to rub myself against you, and you would tell me that you needed me. I would then get on my knees and pull your pants down along with your boxers. I would take your cock in my hand, squeezing it tightly as I started to jerk you off, sucking on your balls a little bit as I did it. I would start off going really slowly, moving my hand up and down your cock really slowly, squeezing it so tight that my nails dug into your skin a little, I would lift my head up so I could suck on your tip, swirling my tongue around it slowly, I would spit on its little bit before I took all of it in my mouth, sucking it up and down really slowly, using my free hand to squeeze at your balls, tugging on them and pulling on them. I would look up at you as I took all of your cock in my mouth, hallowing my cheeks out and then I would start to go faster, bobbing my head up and down really fast and then you'd tell me that you wanted more than just a blow job from me so you'd pull me up and I would crawl back on your lap, pulling my skirt up a little bit to rub myself against your hard cock. I would bounce a little bit against you, my ass slapping against your balls as I did. We would hear the garage opening and quickly have to fix ourselves, assuming it was her, but it was just her younger brother so we would go upstairs to her room, and continue what we were doing in there. Your pants would come back down along with your boxers, and I would slip out of my underwear, rubbing myself against your cock slowly, letting out a couple of moans as I rubbed my clit against you, I would probably get really wet, and you would feel it and tell me that you always knew I was into you back, it was so easy to see because of how wet I was. I would tell you to shut up and just enjoy what you were getting. I would tell you to get a condom, and you'd reach into her bedside table and grab one out, and I would put it on you. I would slide myself down onto you, and you'd let out a moan, telling me how amazing my tight pussy felt around your cock, and I would slowly move up and down on it, grinding myself against you as I did, pressing my ass into your balls. You'd grab onto my hips, pulling me down against you harder and I would start moving fast, slamming myself against you, my ass slapping against your balls as I went down. I would lean down and whisper in your ear that my pussy is so much better than hers will ever be and that your little cock is throbbing, so it's obvious I'm better than she is. I would keep moving up and down quickly, trying to get you really close to cumming. I would slam myself against you, reaching back and grabbing your balls really tight, tugging on them, digging my nails into them a little bit as I continued to fuck you really hard. You'd tell me that you needed to cum, that you were really close. I would tell you to wait, that I wanted to more and that I was gonna let you fuck me until you come inside your condom. So I would lean against her bed, and you would come up behind me and grab my hips and slam your hard throbbing cock into my tight pussy, and you would keep on fucking me until you told me that you needed to cum and I would tell you to beg to cum. You would beg, asking me if you could please cum and finally, after a little bit of denial, I would let you cum inside the condom. You would then pull out and go to the bathroom to clean yourself up, and I would find my panties and put them back on, grabbing the condom package, and I would shove it into my bra, making sure she couldn't find it. You and I would go back downstairs, and you would help me fix my hair so I would look decent and just as we finished fixing ourselves she would walk in and apologize for taking so long and that she hoped we hadn't been too bored while she was gone. She would come and sit in your lap, and I would tell her that we did just fine on our own.

Cheater pt. 2

When her parents were out of town, she would invite us all over to spend the night and probably drink some. I knew that coming tonight might bring up some things from the last time we saw each other and honestly I was kind of hoping for it. We would all be hanging out in her room, playing video games and drinking some beer, she might even invite another guy over for me to talk to. While I was off talking to this guy, you would be watching and probably get a little jealous since you have a little crush on me. We would all play drinking games and watch a couple of movies, and when it was time for bed, she would be knocked out since she is such a lightweight. We would stay up talking until it was very late and you would make a pass at me, leaning over and kissing me, and I would tell you that we couldn't, she's right there and we were bound to get caught. You'd tell me that you didn't care because you missed me and you needed to be with me again like we did last time. I would probably deny you a couple more times, and you would give up and lay down on the floor, and I would lay down next to her on the bed, and after a while of sitting awake, I would reconsider. I would get up and come straddle you, I would lean down and press my lips to yours, and you'd wake up, I would whisper in your ear that I wanted you too, I wanted this right now, and so it would happen. We should start by making out, and I would grind myself against you, you would love the feeling of your cock being rubbed against through your underwear. I would reach down and shove my hand in your boxers, grabbing your cock and jerking it off still inside them as I made out with you. I would squeeze my hand tight around your hard cock, jerking you off really fast, and we would have to be quiet so I would keep my lips on yours the whole time, muffling the moans you let out with your mouth so we wouldn't wake her. You'd mumble against my lips that you wanted to feel my tight pussy again around your cock and I would tell you that I had something a little different in mind to start off. I would go down slowly, kissing along your chest as I made my way down to your cock, I would slowly rub my tongue up your shaft, spitting on the tip and spreading it down your cock as I jerked you off. I would suck on your tip a little bit, continuing to jerk you off, I would use my free hand to play with your balls, squeezing them and tugging on them as I sucked you off. I would then start bobbing my head slowly, taking all of your cock in my mouth, continuing to play with your balls as I sucked on your throbbing cock. I would start to bob my head faster, you'd take a fistful of my hair and start shoving my head down on your cock, and as it hit the back of my throat, I would squeeze your balls really tight. I would then crawl back up and start rubbing myself against you, leaning down to kiss you as I did. You would love the feeling of my undies on your bare hard cock. I would reach into your back

45

pocket and pull your wallet out, grabbing the condom that you kept in it, using my teeth to rip it open, pushing it down over your cock. I would push my panties aside and lip my hips a little bit so I could ease myself down on your cock. I would start off slow, pressing my hips into yours, my ass grinding against your balls as I did, I would slowly move up and down on your cock, I would lean down and kiss your lips really softly, letting out small moans as I fucked you. You would tell me how much you hated wearing condoms with me, how much you just wanted to feel how wet my pussy was when I fucked you. I would tell you to be quiet, that you probably never be able to feel that, especially since you're with my best friend. I would get pissed a little because I was starting to become jealous of her so I would start going up and down quicker, slamming myself down against your cock, my ass slapping against your balls as I did. I would sit up a little bit as I did, shoving my index and middle finger in your mouth so you would be quiet. My other hand would be working on your balls, squeezing them and tugging on them as I fucked you really hard. I would start grinding my hips into yours, and you'd tell me that you needed to cum and I would tell you to wait a little bit before you did. I would try my best to make myself cum, but it wouldn't be enough for me so I would just let you cum in the condom. I would tell you that I wanted to cum, that you should eat me out so I could. I would lay back, and you would dip your head down and start eating me out, I would have to cover my mouth so I wouldn't moan and you would stick a couple of fingers inside me as you sucked on my clit a little bit and then I would cum, and you'd feel my pussy getting tighter as I did and you would lick it all up and then I would tell you to go discard of the condom and to enjoy this cause it wasn't gonna happen again. I would crawl back into bed beside her, curling up next to her after I had just fucked her boyfriend. In the morning when it was time to go I would catch her kissing you, and all that would go through my mind is how the last time your lips were on something it was my pussy, and she tasted it on your lips.

Bad Husband!

It would be around the holidays, a little bit before Christmas when families are visiting each other. You would come over to my house with your wife, my sister; you'd be staying for a couple of days. We would all have a dinner together, me my husband my sister and you would all be sitting around together just talking about how our lives had been, what we were up to and any kind of drama we could think of. You would keep looking at me during dinner, and I would probably look back as well, you were very attractive, much more attractive than the man I was with. I couldn't help but be jealous of my sister, how she always got the better life, hotter husband, bigger house, nicer job, I wanted to take something from her, kind of even the scores. After dinner, you two would go back to your room, and I would be in mine, I would hear you get up and go downstairs for some water, and I would probably follow you, an idea in mind. I would find you in the kitchen in just your boxers, your hair kinda messy and your glasses kinda crooked, sipping on a glass of water. I would immediately cover myself since I was just in my underwear and a tank top, my hair pulled up messily I would clear my throat and say I was just there to get some water and you would kinda back away, and I would fill up my cup, leaning against the counter as I sipped on it. You would be across from me, and I would catch you looking at me, I can't say I wasn't enjoying it. You would quickly look away and apologize; I would tell you that it was totally fine. I would finish my drink and set it down in the sink and hope that as I walked away, you would say something to me, and sure enough, you did. You would tell me that you had been thinking of me ever since dinner, how you could not get over how cute I was to you, and how bad you wanted to bang me, just once at least, even though you were with my sister. I would furrow my eyebrows a little as if I was thinking about your offer when I reality in my head I had already said yes about a million times. I would nod a little bit, taking your hand and dragging you into the living room, I would push you down against the couch, crawling into your lap so I could grind myself against you, pressing my lips to yours as I did. You would buck your hips up against mine, and I would keep pushing mine back down against yours. You would tell me that I was so much hotter than my sister and for some odd reason that would turn me on. I would keep rubbing myself against you as your cock got even harder for me, I would then get down on my knees, pulling your cock through the little slot in your boxers and I would start jerking you off, you would lean your head back and enjoy it as I sucked you off, bobbing my head up and down slowly, looking up at you as I did. I would squeeze your balls tightly as I sucked you off, taking all of your cock in my mouth, gagging a little bit as it hit the back of my throat, my eyes would tear up a little bit, and you would tell me that you wouldn't last much longer like this so I would get back up and sit in your lap, rubbing myself against you a little bit more before I pushed my panties aside and slid myself down against you and you would moan out my name, grabbing my hips and pushing me down against your cock. I would slam myself down against you, and you would tell me that I am ten times better than your wife ever was, and I would tell you your cock was better than my husbands. I would grind myself down against you as I fucked you, slamming my ass against your balls and I would dig my nails into your shoulders, leaning my head down into your neck, kissing on it a little bit and then I would suck on it softly, moving my hips up and down really fast on your cock, and you would tell me you were really close to cumming and I would get off of you and lean down so I could suck you off, tugging on your balls and pulling at them, squeezing them until I let you cum in my mouth. I would wipe my mouth off and tell you that I had a good time, and maybe it could happen again next time we saw each other.

Bad Baby Boy

It would be a Saturday night visiting one of the friends I hadn't seen in a while, we would all be laughing and having a good time, and I would think things were going really great. We would be drinking, probably talking about dumb shit her and I used to do in the past, and we would all be enjoying ourselves. I would excuse myself getting up to go to the bathroom. I would give you a kiss before I walked away. I wouldn't notice, but you would get a boner as you watched me walk to the bathroom, staring at how amazing my ass looked in the dress I was wearing. I would quickly return, noticing that you and she were laughing a lot about something and she would reach over and touch your arm, and I would notice that your pants were a little tight around your crotch area, showing that you had a hard-on. I would be pissed because you didn't even deny her attention, you were feeding into it, enjoying it and I would clear my throat, and you would look up at me and give me a little look like "I'm so sorry." but that would be it for me I would get so mad, but I would play it off like we had to go. I would tell you to get our stuff, and I would walk outside and start the car, you would follow behind me and ask what was wrong and I would ignore you, pulling out of the driveway and heading towards our house. The drive would be silent, and you would reach to turn the radio on, and I would smack your hand away and give you a death glare, and you would just sit back in your seat and be quiet until you noticed that we weren't on our way home anymore, I had taken a street that headed away from it and you would ask me where we were going, and I would just tell you we needed to make a stop before we got home. I would keep driving for another good 15 minutes before I stopped the car and I parked it on the side of the road. I would tell you to get in the back seat and wait for me there. I would probably sit in the front for a little bit, texting people and just ignoring you until I was ready to come back there myself. I would climb in the back, and you would ask me what I was doing and why I was so mad, I would probably clench my jaw and just smash my hand against your cock, you'd let out a loan groan and ask me what that was for and I would just say earlier. I would push you down against the seat, the back of your head barely missing the side of the door, it would hit the cushion with a thud, and I would slip out of my panties, shoving them in your mouth and telling you to stay fucking quiet, I was gonna use you until I was done and if you tried to stop me, it would go on for longer. I would slowly unbutton and unzip your nice little khaki pants, pulling them down slowly, pushing them to the floor. I would then start to unbutton your shirt, slowly going from one button to the next, I would slowly drag my nails down your chest, leaving scratch marks in my wake that would probably be there for a couple of days. I would tell you to put your hands above your head; I didn't want you to touch me right now cause

I was disgusted with you and the only reason why I'm doing this is that I'm trying to teach you a lesson. I would then trace my cold index finger along your stomach all the way down to your crotch, leaving you with goosebumps all over your body. I would then hook my finger under the elastic of your boxers, pulling it up really far before I let it go and it would slap against your skin, and you would let out a little groan. I would then pull them down slowly as well, rubbing my hand against your already hard cock, pulling it back a couple of times just so I could smash my fist against your cock. I would then take your little cock in my hand and start jerking you off, squeezing my hand around your cock my nails digging into it as I jerked you off, scratching your cock so much it was close to bleeding. I would tell you to spread your legs so I could punish your idiotic self some more. You would listen to me of course; I would push my knee up to your balls, kneeing them really hard you would let out a loud moan, almost crying at the pain I would do it again, probably a couple more times. I would then reach up into the front in the centre console and pull out a condom, slowly putting it on your cock and then I would slowly sit myself down on your tiny cock, I would lean down and whisper in your ear how useless you are, your cock can't even make me feel good, and right now you disgust me, but I'm gonna use you until it hurts. I would slowly fuck you, moving my hips up and down on you, you would be making a lot of noise feeling my tight pussy around your little cock. I would remind you that I am the best you'll ever have and if you even try to find somebody else they will never live up to what I am to you right now. I would turn myself around still on your cock, so my back was faced to you, I would keep moving up and down slowly, holding your balls in my hand, squeezing at them as I fucked you really slowly, trying my best to torture you. I would start hitting your balls repeatedly, just over and over and over again until you could hardly feel them, your cock would be so swollen from the need to cum that you were in tears, begging me through the underwear in your mouth to let you cum. I would then speed up, slamming myself down against your cock, continuing to punch and pull and pinch your balls, you'd tell me that you wanted to cum again and I would say no that you don't deserve that at all right now. I would turn around and spit in your face, hopping off your cock for a little bit so I could put my knee over your balls, pressing all my weight into them, you would bite down on my panties, trying to be as quiet as you could so you wouldn't make me any angrier than I already was. I would slam myself down on your tiny cock, leaning down to whisper how useless you are how worthless you are and how much I hate your tiny little cock how it disgusts me sometimes. I would probably spit in your face again and keep on fucking you, my ass slamming against your balls, grinding my pussy onto you as I did and you would beg to cum, and I would finally let you cum inside the condom, making you get out and discard of it outside. When you got back inside, I would grab your cock again and make you lay back again so I could torture your cock and balls some more. I would slowly rub my knee over your balls and wait for you to get hard so I could press all my weight into them again, bouncing up and down a little, shaking the whole car as I hurt you. You would whine out and tell me how bad it was hurting you, that you wanted me to stop but you didn't really, you were kinda enjoying how much I was hurting you. I would keep on doing it, leaning up to spit in your face and remind you who you are, pushing all my weight into your balls once more before I stopped, brining you really close to cumming before I got out and sat back in the front seat, telling you to hurry up and get in with me. When you did, I would explain to why you received this punishment, and if it happened again, there would be worst. I would tell you that I loved you, and I just get really jealous, so don't go talking to others when especially my friend. You would just nod a little, and I would pull you closer to me and whisper that you were going to be okay, that's I love my baby boy so much even though he acts up sometimes. The only reason why I did this was to remind you of me so you wouldn't be looking at another girl ever again because I am the only women that deserve it. I would tell you that I only went so hard on you because I need you in my life and I can't risk losing you to anybody. I would then reach over and grab you hand and kiss it, driving us both home so we could head to bed now.

Office Fun!

We would both be attending a work Christmas party, and we would both be there with our spouses. We wouldn't really know each other because we worked on different floors. I would be walking around, talking to everybody I knew introducing my husband to them, and he would keep his arm wrapped around my waist. You would probably be at the snack table, getting something to drink for you and your wife and you would see me, in my tight dress that showed off my ass and my tits really well, and you couldn't help but stare, you would find yourself even getting hard over me, just watching as I walked around talking to people. You'd stay there just holding on to the two drinks you were carrying until you snapped out of it and started walking back to your wife with your little boner, just as I was walking towards the snack table we would bump into each other, and you'd probably spill the drink on me, and my leg would brush up against your boner as we collided. I would take a step back immediately, grabbing some napkins from the table and trying to dry myself off, you would start apologizing for a bunch of times, trying to help me dry off, patting down my boobs as you did, causing your cock to get harder. I'd tell you that it was fine, my dress would be fine, but I was worried about the little problem in your pants. You'd get really squirmy because the reason it was there was because of me and you'd nod a little bit, trying to change the subject to what my job was, but I would bring it right back to your boner. I would ask what got you if it was one of the little assistants with their short skirts and constant need to show their availability to everybody in the workspace. You'd just shake your head, and I would try and get a read on you but I couldn't so I would lean in a little closer, whispering softly that maybe I could take care of that for you. I would look down at your cock as I said it, watching it twitch in your pants and that would be enough of an answer for me, I would look around to make sure my husband was occupied, and of course, he was, talking to a little assistant. I would grab you by your collar and drag you out to one of the offices down the halls, closing the door behind us and turning on one of the lamps. I would grab you and pull you closer to me, backing you up towards the deal so you could sit. I would kiss along your jaw slowly up to your lips, brushing them against yours and I pushed myself between your legs, pressing myself into your boner. As I started rubbing my hand against your boner, squeezing it through your pants a little bit you'd tell me that the real reason why you were hard was that you were staring at my body and it made you hard. I would lean back a little bit and furrow my eyes together, parting my lips a little bit before I spoke, telling you that you were a little pervert, staring at another woman with your wife no more than 10 feet away from you. I would then reach my hand down into your pants and grab your cock, pulling it up and out of your pants roughly, squeezing my hand tight around it as I started to jerk you off. I would tug and pull on your cock, being extremely rough with it, leaning in to tell you that I was going be rough with you because you are such a naughty man. I would push all the things off the desk and make you lay back. I would lean down a little bit and start running my tongue up your shaft slowly, spitting on your tip to make it really sloppy, I would jerk you off really fast, my hand squeezing your cock really tight. I would then suck on your tip a little bit, bobbing my head slowly and you would just watch me, I would look up at you as I started to go faster, taking all of your cock in my mouth with ease. I would keep sucking you off quickly until you told me that if I did this for much longer, you'd cum. I would stop, leaning back a little bit so I could pull my panties off, straddling you, I would grind myself against you until I made myself really wet. I would reach down into one of the drawers on the desk, pulling out a condom. You'd ask me how I knew condoms were in there and I would just tell you that it was my bosses office, and I knew. I would rip it open with my teeth, pushing it down on your cock slowly. I would rub your tip against my entrance slowly before I slid down on it. I would start off slowly, moving up and down on your cock, grinding myself into you as I did, my ass moving against your balls. You would tell me how amazing my tight pussy feels around your hard cock, and I would just nod a little bit, leaning down and pressing my lips to yours. I would keep going slow for a while, grinding my wet pussy into your throbbing cock before I couldn't take it anymore. I would start moving my hips up and down quicker, letting out a little moan against your mouth before I sat back up, rubbing my hand over my tit slowly, using the other one to rub against my clit. I would let out a loud moan, slamming myself down against your cock. I would grind myself into you, my ass slapping against your balls as I fucked you. I would then lean down and tell you that you couldn't cum until I did, you would start matching my movements, pushing your hips up as I went down and I would keep on going faster, the desk starting to squeak alittle bit as we did. Once I finally came, I would let out a loud moan, telling you that you could cum. I would reach my hand back, grabbing your balls, squeezing them as I slammed down against you until you come inside your condom. As soon as you finished, I would hop off of you, pulling my panties back up and checking my appearance in the little window. I would tell you that the next time you come to an event and start staring at women and getting hard, to wear darker colour pants because it was very easy to tell. I would then open the door, heading back to you for a second, leaning down and giving you a kiss o the forehead before I walked out of the office, leaving you to clean yourself up. I would walk back to my husband, who was still talking to a little blonde assistant, telling him I spilt something on myself and that I wanted to leave and we would, and you would never find out my name.

Family Matters!

We would we visit my parents for the holidays, and it would be my turn to come to see mine this Christmas. The whole house would smell like food; my mom would probably stressing about her fondue party she does every year, running around trying to make everything perfect. My dad would probably be stuck in a line at Walmart trying to buy something my mom had forgotten. We would be seated on the couch in my living room, probably scrolling through our phones I might be playing a game, and you'd be on porn even after me telling you multiple times not to do that. For a while I would mind my own business, playing my little game on my phone but I would notice that you were squirming around a lot, pulling at your pants and almost hiding what was on your phone from me. You would grab one of the pillows from the couch and put it over your lap, sticking one of your hands under it and I would be very suspicious. I would try and sneakily glance at it as you weren't looking and then I would look down to see a little bulge in your pants, trying my best to give you the benefit of the doubt and I would just think it was the way your pants were situated. You would keep on watching porn, and I would see it, getting pissed off that you were watching porn after I specifically told you not to. I would grab the pillow out of your lap to see you had your hand down your pants I would be furious, doing this kind of shit I my living room. I would give you the death glare and clench my teeth, it would take everything in me not to just punch you in the balls right now, but I wanted to drag it out. I would just grab your phone and set it beside me, pulling a blanket over us and get really close to you so it would look like we were cuddling and I would rest my hand in your lap, pulling your pants down a little so I could pull your cock out along with your balls. I would wrap my hand around your shaft really tight, my nails digging into your skin and you would let out a little groan trying to hold in the noises you wanted to make as I would jerk you off really hard, my nails scraping along your shaft as I did. My parents might come into the living room, and I wouldn't even care, cause I was so angry at you for doing that. I would even slam my fist against your balls, and you'd let out a little noise and my parents would look over at us, and you'd just clear your throat and look back at the tv, and I would continue to do this, telling you that later I was going to do so much to you because you did this. I would jerk you off so fast your cock would throb and I would punch you in the balls until they went numb and you were whispering in my ear begging me to let you cum for me. I would make you wait a little bit, trying to drag this out as much as I could and finally I'd let you cum, and it would get all over your nice dress shirt, and you would have to excuse yourself to go change. Later that night, you would get more because of the fact you weren't listening to me.

Friday Night Fights

It would be a normal night for me; I would probably be in my apartment, unpacking my things, trying to get my life together, or just doing some homework I hadn't gotten around to. It would be very slow for me, barely being able to keep my eyes open because I was so bored. That would change when I started to overhear one of my neighbours fighting, yelling about something I couldn't quite make out. I would stand up and press my ear to the wall, trying to listen in on what it was about because I am nosy, I could make out certain things, something about how the guy was a jerk and how the girl was a bitch. I decided to stop listening in after a little while, sitting back down on my couch. Things would go quiet for a little bit until I heard a loud slam of the door, and I would feel bad. I knew 12 am probably wasn't the best time to introduce myself, but I felt bad, and I wanted to check in on whoever was left. I would check myself in the mirror, fixing myself a little bit before I made my way over to the door, taking in a deep breath before I knocked on the door. I was only in a small tank top, some shorts and my socks, I was kind of regretting coming to meet my new neighbour in this outfit, especially if it was a cute guy. I would shake my head a little bit, biting down on my bottom lip as I heard the door open, a husky voice speaking something about how you knew I would come back to apologize, you stopped speaking as soon as you realized I wasn't who you thought I was. You would look me up and down trying not to laugh at what I was wearing; it was clear you had been drinking, I could smell the alcohol on you. You'd ask who I was and why I was at your apartment and if I was one of your girlfriend's friends trying to test him, it wasn't going to work. I would shake my head, holding my hand out for you to shake as I introduced myself. You would shake my hand, and I would explain that I lived in the next apartment over, and I figured I would introduce myself. You would just nod your head and ask if that was all and I would say yes. I would start to walk away, and you'd grab my arm, pulling me back. You'd tell me that you have had a rough night and you needed somebody to stay with you to keep your mind off of things, or you might do something crazy so I would come inside, looking around at the messy apartment, it was clear the fight had gotten pretty bad, somebody had thrown things around. I would follow behind you as you led me to the living room, taking a seat on your couch. You would sit beside me and grab your beer, taking another sip and I would just sit there awkwardly, trying to think about what to say. You would just look at me, and I would look right back and the next thing I know your empty beer can was on the floor, and you'd lip were on mine. Your lips were cold and tasted disgusting thanks to your beer, your kiss would be sloppy, it was clear you were a bit out of it, but I wouldn't protest, in fact, I kind of liked it. Your hands would cup my cheeks, and I would wrap my arms around your neck, pressing my lips to yours, we would make out for a good 10 minutes before I noticed your boner pressing into my leg. I would push you off a little bit and ask if this was really what you wanted to do, you would just nod and say to keep going. I would trail my fingertips down your chest, grabbing your hard cock through your pants, I would squeeze it a little bit as you kissed on my neck. I would quickly unbutton your pants, pulling the zipper down slowly, trying not to think about how wrong what I was doing was. I would take your cock in my hand, wrapping my hand tightly around it, squeezing it almost as I started to jerk you off, I would move my hand up and down it slowly, rubbing my thumb over your head every so often and you would let out a moan, I would lean down and suck on your tip softly, using my free hand to play with your balls, squeezing them a little bit, I would then take all of your cock in my mouth, wrapping my lips around your throbbing cock, I would start bobbing my head up and down slowly at first, using my hand to jerk odd whatever I couldn't reach. I would look up at you as I did, your hand would be fisted in my hair, watching me as I sucked you off. I would start to go quicker, moving my mouth up and down your cock quickly, my tongue swirling over your tip, gagging slightly as it hit the back of my throat. I would then lift my head up, crawling into your lap, rubbing myself against your cock slowly, pressing myself down into you, you'd grab my hips, encouraging me to do more and I would. I would start bouncing up and down on it, my ass pressing into your balls. I would stand back up; you'd look up at me, watching what I was doing. I would pull my shorts and undies down, letting them fall to the floor. I would then crawl back into your lap, straddling your sides. I would grind my pussy against your cock, leaning down and kissing your neck as I did. My ass would move against your balls, causing your cock to twitch against my wet pussy. I'd ask if you had a condom and you'd reach into your pocket pulling one out; I would take it from you, ripping it open and pushing it down over your cock. I would lift my hips, moving your cock over my entrance a little bit before I sat down on it, letting out a little moan as I did. I would start moving slowly, lifted my hips as I moved up and down, you would grip my hips, trying to get me to move faster and I would shake my head, trying to drag this out as long as I could. I would move up and down, grinding my pussy into you as I did, my ass moving against your balls. After a while of doing that I would start to go faster, you'd lean your head back letting out a loud moan. I would slam myself against you, and you would tell me how much you loved my tight pussy around your throbbing cock. I would reach back and grab your balls as I fucked you, grinding myself into you as I moved up and down quickly on you. You'd tell me that you were about to cum when you would hear a faint knocking at the door. I would stop dead in my tracks, and I would hop off of you, asking who that was. You'd tell me it was probably your girlfriend and that you were gonna hide me somewhere. I would grab my shorts and put them back on, following you to your closet and I would stay in there quietly, waiting for you to come back. When you finally returned a good 30 minutes later, you'd tell me that we could finish this another time, that you had to sneak me out of here. I would follow behind you in the dark, looking over and seeing your girlfriend asleep in your bed and then I would step out into the hallway. You'd lean out and tell me to come closer; you'd whisper in my ear a thank you, telling me that you were glad you weren't alone tonight and that you hoped to see me again. I would nod a little bit turning to walk away when you would grab my arm and tell me to give you a kiss. I would roll my eyes and lean up to give you a small kiss on the lips.

So We Meet Again

I would probably be in my room, sitting on my couch when I would hear a pounding against the wall, followed by some moans. I would roll my eyes, knowing you and your girlfriend were up for another round of makeup sex. I would turn my TV up, trying my best to focus on what was on. I would give up when I couldn't hear over her constantly screeching your name. I would head to my bathroom, stepping in the shower to try and drown it out. I wished paper-thin walls was listed as one of the features when I was looking at this apartment. After I finished showering, I would get dressed and sit back down in my living room, thanking God you two had shut up. I would decide to go for a walk, just as I was heading out you'd be heading out too. You would walk out just as I was coming down the hall and I would accidentally bump into you, dropping my keys. I would bend down and get them, standing back up and looking you in the eyes. We would kinda just stand there for a while, looking at each other before I broke the silence. I would tell you that next time you and your girlfriend decided to go for a new record of how many times you can fuck in a night to put a muzzle on her.

You'd laugh a little and shake your head, making a smart come back on how I could join you for one more round if I wanted. I would be tempted, asking if your girlfriend was still there and you would say no. I would chew at my bottom lip, playing with the ring on my finger deciding on whether or not it was worth it, I would think back to the last time we did something and how you never finished and how bad I felt. After a lot of thinking and overthinking, I would finally agree, pushing you back into your apartment, shutting the door behind me with my foot. I would keep pushing you back, headed towards your room. I would push you down against the bed, letting my hair down as I crawled on top of you, telling you how I had been waiting for the opportunity to finish what we started. I would lean down and kiss against your neck, grinding myself against you slowly until you got really hard for me. I would pull your pants down a little, taking your cock in my hand and jerking you off, my hand would be tight around it my nails scraping your shaft as I jerked you off really fast. I would use my free hand to grab your balls, pulling on them and tugging on them. I would stand back up to slip out of my pants and underwear, leaning down to suck on your cock a little bit. I would non my head up and down quickly, looking up at you, squeezing your balls as I sucked you off. I would do that for a little while before crawling back on top of you. I would to myself against you, telling you that this time we won't be interrupted. You would nod a little bit as I am grinding myself against you, my ass moving against your balls slowly. I would move up and down on it, slamming myself against it, putting all my weight on your cock. I would then lift my hips a little, rubbing my pussy against your tip slowly before I slid down on it. I would let outs loud moan, starting off slowly as I fucked you so you could feel every inch of my tight pussy wrapped around your throbbing cock. I would grind myself into you as I went down, reaching back and playing with your balls as I did. I would start to go faster, moving up and down quickly on your cock. You would grip at my hips, telling me how much better I am than your girlfriend. I would slam myself against you, my ass slapping against your balls as I did. I would lean down as I slammed my hips against yours, grinding myself into you, I would press my lips to yours, kissing on your jawline as well. You'd tell me that you were close so I would get off of you, getting into my knees, taking your cock in my hand and looking up at you as I jerked you off quickly. I would lean down a little to suck on your balls some, leaning back and opening my mouth wide to let you cum in my mouth, swallowing all of it as soon as you did. I would grab my things heading towards the door, figuring my work here was done. You'd call me back for a second, telling me that you were glad we ran into each other again, hoping to do it again soon. I would agree, reminding you about the muzzle for your girlfriend, as I headed down the hall I would pass your girlfriend heading back to your apartment with food or something, thanking god we finished in time.

Bonus Baby

It would be a normal Tuesday morning for you, the same routine you went through every day, get up in the morning, get ready for your day at work, grab a coffee for you and your boss, trying to suck up for a nice bonus, get to work, do your work and go home. It wouldn't go down that way at all today; you were in for a big treat after you found out it brought your kid to the workday. Now you, you didn't have any kids at the time so you were just sitting in your office as per usual, typing in numbers to the computer when you would like me, a small younger blonde who was a fresh face. You'd never seen me around before; you'd wonder if she was new, glad that something different was happening. I would make my way around the small office, watching as everybody did their work, pretending to care to make my father happy. I would walk past your little cubicle area, looking over your things and getting excited when I saw a little toy Yoda sitting on your desk, telling you that I loved Star Wars. You'd nod a little, and we would talk for a while, I'd grow a little soft spot for you, wondering if you could be into what I was. I would start hinting at it, that I wanted to do something with you. After a while of you not getting it I would flat out ask you, "If you let me do something with you, I can get you that bonus you've been dying for." you'd nod a little bit, having to think over what on earth I could want with you, but you'd agree to it, I was hot, and you needed the money. I would take you to one of the empty conference rooms, locking it behind me and closing up the windows. I would smile a little bit, telling you to lay back on the table. I would pull your pants down, along with your boxers, watching as your cock popped out, already hard from God knows what, you would be shocked at first, not at all expecting this out of me at all. I would quickly grab your cock, jerking you off really hard, my hand squeezed tight around your shaft, my nails digging into the skin. You'd tell me that it was hurting and I would tell you that if you wanted that promotion, you'd let me continue. I would lean down, taking your cock in my mouth, using my free hand to squeeze on your balls, I would kind of scrape my teeth along your shaft as I sucked you off, you would tell me that it was hurting you and I would tell you to suck it up, this is nothing compared to what I wanted to do. I was hoping to get me a cute older man at my daddy's work, hoping to do what I wanted with him, making him feel like he's a little boy again, my property to use and abuse. I would stop after a little while, going back to jerking you off really hard. I would crawl on top of you, wedging my knee in between your legs, leaning down to kiss you below ear before I spoke telling you that you were my little boy now, and everything that I do you will end up liking even though it will hurt again. I would rub my knee over your balls slowly, pulling your tie up and shoving it in your mouth before I put my weight into them. You would cry out a little bit, not used to this, but when I was done, you'd be begging for more. I would kiss your cheek softly, telling you that I was gonna take care of you. I would pull my weight off of them, rubbing them softly with my hands before I started putting more weight on them. I would kiss you to get you to shut up, not wanting anybody to find us in here or you would get fired. I would move my weight around on them as you cried out, I would tell you to be a good boy for me, to stop being a baby and crying. I would then press all my weight into them, letting out a little moan as I did because it turned me on so much. I would reach my hand down and jerk your cock off as I kept on pressing all of my weight into your little balls. I would tell you that you were doing good my little boy, that soon it would be over when I let you finally cum. I would tell you to jerk yourself off as I did this last bit. I would rest both my hands on your thighs, watching as you jerked yourself off, I would dig my hands in before I lifted all my weight up and then smashed it back down. You'd beg me to cum, and after you asked nicely, I would tell you that you could. You'd be jerking yourself off as I smashed my weight into your balls and you'd release onto your nice work shirt. I would then get up and tell you that you were a good boy, very sick but good. I would keep up with my end of the bargain, telling my father that you deserved a bonus, I saw how hard you worked, and he would give it to you.

Busted

I would probably be away for the night maybe with friends, and you and my son would be hanging out, you might invite a few girls and you would all be doing stuff, probably smoking and drinking as most young teens do. I would come back home probably a little tipsy cause we were drinking, and when I would see you all had girls over I would get pretty upset for you guys doing this without my permission I would make the girls leave and as soon as they did I would be yelling at my son and also at you, getting mad that you allowed it. I would tell you both that I was very disappointed in you. I would send you back to my son's room, coming in there and finding all the stuff, I would gather up all the alcohol and the remaining weed. I would take it back to my room and slam the door shut. You would come to find me in my room and apologize for doing that, that you and my son knew better and you took advantage of me being gone. I would probably still be pretty tipsy, so I would get really mad, and I would push you up against the wall and tell you to shut your mouth. I would shove my knee between your legs and push it up against your balls, and you would start apologizing more and more, and I would cover your mouth with my hand. I would shove my knee into your balls, and you would cry out into my hand, and it would muffle it. I would tell you to shut up so my son couldn't hear us, if you wanted to make it up to me you would have to do this for me. I would reach down and grab your cock, stroking it slowly as I jammed my knee into your balls again, you would double over, and I would straighten you back up again, making sure you kept your back to the wall. I would take my hand off your mouth to kiss you, telling you that I wanted you to do the work now, that I wanted you to slam your balls against my leg until it hurt so bad you felt pleasure like never before. I was gonna show you how much better an older woman could be, rather than a scrawny inexperienced teen girl. I would jerk your cock off as you started pushing yourself down on my knee. I would keep telling you it wasn't good enough every time you did it; I'd tell you how pathetic and weak you were, that you should be a man. You'd start slamming yourself down against me, whimpering every time you did, and you would be getting closer to how hard I wanted you to do it, I would pull your cock up, pushing you down against me even harder, I would bury my face in your neck, kissing on it as you slammed yourself against me, it would make me really wet, listening to your pain, it oddly turning me on. I would grab you by your collar and drag you over to the bed where I would slam you down against it, crawling on top of you and rubbing myself against you slowly. I would bounce against your throbbing cock, grinding my pussy against it, letting out a moan as my clit rubbed against you. I would push my panties aside, slamming myself down against your cock. You'd let out a moan as you felt my tight pussy wrapping around your throbbing cock. I would start out slow, moving my hips up and down, rolling my hips into you, I would grind my ass against your balls, digging my nails into your chest as I fucked you. After a while of doing that I would go faster, slamming myself down against you, my ass slapping against your balls, your cock would start twitching inside me, and you'd tell me that you were close to cumming. I would tell you to wait a little bit until I was ready. I would reach back and squeeze your balls as I fucked you, grabbing your hand and placing it over my breast, telling you to touch me more. I would keep fucking you, my pussy rubbing against your cock as I rode you. I would then hop off of you, taking your cock in my hand, my knee hovering over your balls. I would start jerking you off really fast, pressing all of my weight into your balls as you did. It would hurt you at first, but you would grow to enjoy it more and more. I'd keep pumping your cock in my hand, pressing my weight on your balls as I did, my hand tight around your shaft, my nails digging in. You'd beg me to let you cum, that if you held it in any longer, you might explode. I finally would tell you that you could cum and as I did you would cum all over your stomach. I would make you clean up and go back to my son's room, and you'd have to lay next to the boy whose mom just fucked you.

Wedding Bells

It's my wedding day; I would be getting ready to marry the man that I loved with all my heart. I would be getting ready for the wedding, my makeup would be done perfectly, and my hair would be up and looking amazing. I will have just gotten into the most beautiful wedding dress ever made; it would fit me perfectly, making me look really good. You would walk in and stop in your tracks, just staring at me and you would breathe a little harder, looking at me up and down, and you would tell me how amazing I looked. I would probably blush a little and say thank you and get a little nervous cause I always thought you were cute, even though you were my soon to be husbands best friend. You'd walk over to me and brush a piece of hair out of my face and tell me that I was beautiful and that I better treat your best friend right, or else. I would ask you what you were talking about, and you'd tell me if we broke up you wouldn't be very happy with me. I would ask who you thought you were, coming in here and threatening me. I would push you back against the wall, my body would be pressed up against yours, and I would look up into your eyes and furrow my eyebrows, and you would brush your hand over my cheek and then I would lean up and kiss you. I knew it was wrong; I was about to get married, and here I was kissing his best friend, but honestly, I kinda liked it.

We would make out for a while; I would reach my hand down and feel you up through your suit pants until you were really hard for me. I would pull you back to the little sofa in the corner, pushing you down on it and I would lift my dress, sitting down on your lap. I would rub myself against you, making you even harder; your cock would be throbbing against me. I would tell you that this was really naughty that we were doing this when my husband was just down the hall. Your cock would twitch a little against me, I would move down and pull your pants down, taking your cock in my hand and I would jerk you off slowly, squeezing it as I pumped you, my nails digging into you as I did. I would suck on your tip a little, looking up at you, I would start sucking you off, you would grab the back of my head, pushing my head down as I sucked you off, ruining my perfect hair, I would take all of your cock in my mouth, letting it hit the back of my throat, and I would gag a little, my eyes tearing up making my mascara run and my makeup would be ruined. I would then stand back up, getting in your lap and I would move my brand new panties aside, that happened to be soaked so I could slide down on your cock. I would start off slowly, movingly tight pussy up and down on your cock, grinding myself against you slightly as I went down. I would tell you how much better you are than he is, I would keep moaning out your name. I would then go faster, slamming myself against you, my ass slapping against your balls and I would dig my nails into your chest, my head falling back as I rode you really fast. I would reach back and grab your balls, squeezing them a little bit. You'd tell me you were close and I would get off, leaning down to suck you off, I would jerk you off really fast, sucking on your balls and before I could take your cock in my mouth you would cum on my face. You'd fix yourself and leave as fast as possible, and I would have to fix my makeup along with my hair because I knew it was almost time. After I finished getting myself together I would walk out, and get married to him, glancing over at you every once in a while as I recited my vows, you would wink, and I and I would blush, glancing down and noticing that your fly wasn't all the way up, praying nobody would notice that the both of us weren't really looking as well as we could.

Bad Brother

We would all be over at your parent's house for the holidays at a dinner that the whole family was invited to. We would all be talking about how soon the wedding was and how proud everybody was of your brother, and he would have his hand wrapped around my waist, kissing me and touching me, and I would be showing my ring off, telling everybody how happy I was and how much I loved him. You would be watching from afar, getting jealous of him and how hot is fiancé was. We would sit down for dinner, and you'd be across from me, and you'd keep staring at me, watching me. I would keep catching you looking at me, and I would smile a little bit. You'd start kicking your foot against mine, and I would give you a look to stop, glancing over at your brother to tell you not now. I would excuse myself, going to the kitchen to get some more to drink, you would follow behind me and tell me how great I look and how it's been a long time since we've seen each other. I would nod, trying to get my drink and get back to your brother, but you would stop me, saying that I wasn't going anywhere. You'd pull me aside, trying to kiss me and at first, I would fight it, saying I needed to be faithful to your brother, that this wasn't going to happen. I would eventually give in, letting your lips touch mine. We would make out for a little bit, my leg rubbing up against your cock and you would get really hard for me, loving the fact that somebody could walk in here at any second. You'd pull us over to the closet, reaching your hand down into my pants, moving your fingers against me to make me really wet. I would push my hand down into your pants, grabbing your cock and wrapping my hand around it really tight, digging my nails into it as I jerked you off. I would pull your pants down, getting down on my knees and taking your cock in my mouth, looking up at you as I sucked you off. I would squeeze my hands around your balls, taking all your cock in my mouth, gagging a little bit as I did. You'd tell me that you were gonna cum if I kept doing that. I would stand back up, making you sit down and I would crawl on top of you, sliding down on your cock, letting out a small moan as I did. I would put my hand over my mouth, and I bounced up and down on it. You would tell me how amazing I feel, how tight I am and how lucky your brother is to have me. I would keep moaning into my hand, trying my best to keep quiet as I fucked you. I would start going faster, slamming myself down against you, my ass slapping against your balls. I would grind myself against you as I went down on you. I would dig my nails into your chest, moving my ass against your balls. I would get off of you, taking your cock in my hand and jerking you off, I would lean down sucking on your tip. You would force my head down on your cock as you came in the back of my throat. I would stand back up, swallowing it and hurrying back to my husband, making sure to grab a drink on my way back, kissing him and saying I got distracted. You would return a while after me, making an excuse that you got sick, probably too much to drink. We would both keep our mouths shut about what happened, never talking about it ever.

My Husband's Best Buddie

It would be the night before Christmas, and you would invite your best friend over for dinner with you and your wife, and I would also come because he was my husband. We had never met before, and we most likely would never see each other again. I would be dressed in a really tight black dress, with a nice pair of heels on and I would look really amazing. We would arrive a little early; my husband was always big on being on time. As soon as I walked in you wouldn't be able to keep your eyes off of me, your wife would probably notice, but you didn't care, it was usually of you to stare, but never want somebody this bad. Your cock would already get really hard because of me, poking through a little bit in your pants. We would all sit down around your table, asking why you didn't spend Christmas with family, and you'd tell us that they couldn't make it out this year, they got snowed in. We would all eat and talk about work and other things, how my husband and I were planning to have children soon, hoping to get started because we didn't wanna be really old parents. I would excuse myself, going to the bathroom for a minute, you would go to the kitchen, and on my way back I would bump into you, making you drop what you had in hand and I would help you clean it up. We would both go back to the kitchen, our hands brushing as we put stuff away, I would start to pull back, and you would grab my hand, confessing that ever since you saw me, you knew you had to have me, at least just once. I would get kind of angry at your forwardness, pushing you back against the counter and telling you that you're a sick bastard for wanting to cheat on your wife when she's just out the room. I would wedge my knee up between your legs, pushing it up so far it barely touched the bottom of your balls, I would reach my hand down, squeezing your cock in my hand tightly, rolling my eyes and telling you how disgusting it is that you were already hard, just thinking about me. I would tell you that you were going to regret ever saying something to me because I never normally do this because I love my husband dearly, but I feel like it's something you deserve. I would reach my hand in your pants quickly, grabbing your cock and tightening my hand around it, squeezing it tightly and starting to jerk you off. I would then use my free hand to cover your mouth, knowing the noise you were gonna make would be loud as soon as I did what I would next. I would then shove my knee so far up into your balls, so hard it felt like you may vomit. I would keep jerking you off, my nails digging into your cock as I did. I would keep shoving my knee into your balls, whispering in your ears how gross and perverted and disgusting you are, and it would just

83

make you even harder. I would look into the other room, making sure my husband wasn't getting too cosy with your wife. I would speed it up, starting to jerk your cock off even faster, pounding my knee into your balls but it wouldn't be enough. I would whisper in your ear that I wanted you to do it to yourself, smash your balls down against my knee and make yourself cum as you touched your cock in your pants. I would let go of your cock, watching as you pushed it back into your pants, zipping them back up. You would rub your cock a little bit as you weakly pushed yourself down on my knee, I would tell you to go harder and you would, going a little harder each time but not enough. I would grab your shoulders and dig my nails in, pushing you so far down and so fast you'd only manage to get a little whimper out. You'd keep on doing it as your played with yourself, and I would just watch as you did until finally after a couple of times of you begging me to let you cum I would let you, right in your pants. I would grab the new tray of things you wanted to bring out, setting it down on the table and kissing my husband softly as I started talking to your wife and him. You'd need a second to recover and clean yourself up, but you would then join us again, continuing dinner with your sore cock and cum filled underwear.

Best Friends
Flirty Boyfriend

We would be going to the same high school but never really crossed paths because of our different schedules. One day my best friend would come to me and tell me she had a new boyfriend and I would ask to meet you, and at lunch, we would all sit together, and I would think you're a pretty decent guy, not bad looking so I would give my approval. After lunch, we would all leave and go our separate ways, off to our next class. Later on, as we were switching classes I would notice you in the hallway, obviously flirting with another girl and I would get really pissed off, coming up to you and asking what you were doing, talking to another girl when you were dating my best friend. I would tell the other girl to run off and get to class because I was gonna take care of you. I would pull you into one of the janitor's closets, locking it behind us and slamming you up against the door. I would grab you by your shirt collar asking why you thought it would be okay for you to do that when my best friend likes you so much. You would stammer to get words out, and I would just get even more made, telling you to shut your mouth before I made you. I would push you back against the door again, shoving my knee between your thighs, the back of your head hitting the door a little as I did. I would push my knee up into your crotch asking you again, what you thought you were doing and you would struggle to get the words out because you were nervous about what I might do to you. I would look you in the eye, pressing my knee up even more as you answered me quickly that you were just dumb and that it would never happen again that you were so so sorry. I would just roll my eyes and shove my knee up into your crotch; you would let out a loud groan as my kneecap hit the bottom of your balls, shoving them up into you. I would push you back up again, so you were standing up straight and looking me in my eyes. I would tell you that what you did would never happen again, and what I was gonna do was going to ensure that. I would make you pull your pants down a little bit, taking your cock in my hand, wrapping my hand around it tightly, my nails digging into your shaft. I would start jerking you off really fast, my knee moving up against your balls again, making you confused because it hurt so bad, but it also felt so good, you'd let out another groan, doubling over, I would just dig my nails into your cock, even more, making you stand back up. Your cock would get really sore really fast, starting to throb as I jerked you off. I would keep shoving my knee into your balls, making your balls start to hurt really bad. I would make you sit down in a chair, pushing your legs apart so I could rest my knee on your balls, jerking your cock off really fast. I would lean my weight into your balls, making you cry out, I would tell you to shut it, or it would hurt even worse. I would keep jerking you off as I pressed my weight into you, moving my knee around on your balls slowly. You'd tell me that it hurt so bad and you wanted me to stop, but I would tell you that you needed to learn your lesson, so you would never hurt my best friend. I would then jerk you off even faster, spitting in your face as I slammed my knee into your balls. It would push you over the edge; you'd tell me that you were close to cumming and I would bring you even closer, leaning down and spitting on your cock, using both of my hands to jerk you off slowly, pressing my weight into your balls and as soon as I told you you could cum you would, all over your nice little shirt. I would grab my bag off the floor, starting to leave, I would look back at you telling you if that ever happened again, the next time would hurt worse than this did, and I would give you the sweet release of cumming. I would quickly exit the little closet, making my way to my next class, leaving you there to clean yourself up before you had to see my best friend.

Where Dreams Come True

It would be spring break and my friends, and I had finally gotten to Disney after saving up for so long to go there. It would probably be early in the morning when we arrived, we were excited and wanted to spend as much time as we could there. Once we got in immediately, we would start going on rides, trying to get through as many as we could before the big crowds came in. It would get a little hot, so we might stop for some ice cream. We would be sitting down, enjoying the little break we had before we started going again. Of course, being as clumsy as I am I would probably get ice cream all over my shirt, I would try my best to get everything out, and then one of your friends would come over, offering to help me with that. I would probably accept his help, deciding just to take the shirt off altogether, in the end, just wearing a tank top after it. He would obviously be flirting with me, telling me how pretty I was, rob ably dying inside cause he touched my boob a little while helping me. Then, I would see you. You were walking over with the rest of your friends; you all were wanting to go on another ride. Your friend would still be talking to me, trying to get me to come along with you guys but I would be much more interested in you. When it was time for you guys to go, I would suggest that my friends and I came along with you, hoping to get some time alone with you. We would head over to the haunted mansion, waiting patiently in line for us to get on. You and I would exchange a few glances, and when we got up to the loading area we would end up in the ride together, your friend pretty bummed out that I wasn't with him, but I didn't care. We would make small talk, but there was an obvious tension between us, I mean I could tell you thought exactly what I was. So while the ride started and we were a couple of minutes in I would make my move. I would slowly reach my hand across your lap, slowly pressing my palm into your cock, feeling if you were hard, and you would be just a little bit. I would scoot closer to you, leaning in to whisper in your ear that I knew you wanted it too. I would squeeze your cock tightly through your pants, rubbing my hand over your cock until you were really hard. I would then reach my hand down your pants, taking your cock in my hand and stroking you slowly, my hand wrapped tight around your shaft. I would use my free hand to squeeze your balls, leaning my head down to suck on your tip. I would bob my head up and down slowly, jerking you off in my hand quickly as I did. I would keep squeezing your balls, taking all of your cock in my mouth as I did, your cock would hit the back of my throat, and you'd be enjoying every second of it, knowing that anybody could probably see us doing this, but that would just turn you on even more. You would rest your hand on the back of my head, pushing my head down a little as I sucked you off. I would keep bobbing my head, squeezing your balls tight in my hand. I knew the ride would be ending soon, so I sped it up. I would continue to bob my head quickly, my mouth wrapped tight around your cock, using my hand to jerk you off as I did, my other hand squeezing your balls so tight my nails kinda dug in. My teeth would scrape against your shaft slightly, and you'd buck your hips up into my mouth, telling me you were about to cum and if nod my head, letting you know you could. You would cum in the back of my throat, and I would swallow all of it, wiping my mouth just before the ride ended. We would exit together, spending the rest of the day together with our friends, maybe even exchanging information before it was time to leave. Your friend would be kinda pissed you stole me away from him, asking what the hell you did to make me as you and you'd just laugh it off, keeping our little secret to yourself.

Whipped Cream Cocksicle

It would probably be a late night, we would be up until late talking and just joking around, and I would probably get hungry, and I would drag you downstairs along with me, begging you to make me some ice cream. I would sit on the counter patiently waiting for it, you'd bring it to me, and when you showed up without whipped cream on it, I would just have to get up and get it myself. I would lean down, searching for it in the fridge when I would finally pull it out and spray it on top of my ice cream. I would then tell you to open your mouth, spraying it inside. You would try and swallow it all, but some would drop out of your mouth, landing on your chest, since you weren't wearing a shirt I would just lick it off of you, going back to eating my ice cream, after I finished, I would dump my bowl in the sink, grabbing the whipped cream again, spraying some in my mouth and then going to kiss you, getting it all over you. I'd tell you that I had an idea, but it might get a little sticky. I would pull you over towards the couch, pushing you down on top of it. I would pull your pants and underwear off slowly, tossing them aside. I'd grab the whipped cream again, spraying little dots down your chest, down towards your cock stopping a little bit before it. I would then start licking the whipped cream off of you, really slowly, giving you sloppy kisses all down your chest and to your stomach, my tongue trailing down your abdomen until I stopped at your cock, taking the whipped cream and spraying it over your cock, looking up at you as I slowly licked every bit of it off of your cock. I would then take your cock in my mouth, wrapping my lips around you, slowly bobbing my head, your cock already getting harder and harder until you were throbbing in my mouth. I would use my hand to jerk off the rest of your cock, leaning my head down a little to suck on your balls. I would keep jerking you off quickly, making sure to keep eye contact with you. I would then take your cock back in my mouth, taking all of it in, squeezing your balls in my free hand as I sucked you off. I would keep moving my head up and down quickly, gagging a little as the tip hit the back of my throat, I would look up at you as I did. I would dig my nails into your balls a little as I squeezed them so hard, you would tell me that if I kept this up, you'd be finished soon. I could feel you throbbing in my mouth, twitching a little bit as I took all of your cock in. I would nod a little bit, telling you to cum. You would finally cum in my mouth after I sucked you off for a few more minutes, I would swallow all of it. We would clean up any mess that was leftover, heading back upstairs to bed and I would tell you that you taste ten times better than that whipped cream

Frat House

It would be a Friday night; everybody was ready to kick off the weekend and let some steam off after a long week of lectures and tests. Everybody was going to a big frat house for the big party, lots of booze and drugs and girls in tight short dresses with boys praying they get laid, you being one among them. I would have been there for a while, probably pretty tipsy and trying my best to head out, already sick of the party atmosphere. I would push my way through the big crowd of people heading towards the door, but I would get stopped by drunk guys coming on to me, trying to touch my ass and get me into the nearest room possible. You'd notice I was in a little bit of distress, not knowing I was fully capable of handling myself as most men assume, you came over and tried to help me out, making me only more pissed. I'd grab you by your light coloured polo shirt, pulling you closer to me so you could hear you when u told you I didn't need dumb boys to help and that since you believed I was some helpless girl in danger, I would show you just how much a girl can do to a man. I'd punch my fingers on your ear, dragging you to the closest bedroom I could find, pushing you inside and closing the door behind me. I would push you down on to the bed, slowly pulling the shirt over my head, and tossing it beside me, walking towards you. You'd be sitting up on the bed, just watching me and not knowing what to say. I would then climb into your lap and straddle your legs; I would wrap my arms around your neck, leaning in close to your face, telling you that this would be the best night of your life and you wouldn't even be taking your cock out. I would then start grinding myself against you slowly, your cock starting to get hard for me already. I would tell you to touch my boobs, not letting you be the only one to feel good out of this. I would rub myself against you, our jeans rubbing against each other, creating friction between us. Your cock would start to hurt a little, being constricted by your pants, you'd ask if you could take them off and I would, of course, tell you no, but you already knew that answer. I would keep grinding myself against you, my pussy rubbing against your cock through the fabric, and you would love how it felt. I would start bouncing up and down a little, my ass slapping against your balls as I did, you'd grab my hips, trying to make me go faster but then I would just stop, starting to grind again. I'd tell you that you weren't in charge tonight and I was going to be doing all the work. I would then start bouncing again, slamming myself down against your throbbing cock, making you ache a little more every time I went down. You'd tell me you were close, figures you'd finish early, just a little frat boy who can't last long enough to please a girl. I would start bouncing faster, my ass slamming down against your balls, my pussy rubbing against your cock. I'd make you beg to cum, making you beg for me to let you have some sort of release. After a few minutes, I would finally let you cum, right there in your pants, making a big mess all over yourself. I would then stand up, putting my shirt back on and walking towards the door, reminding you that this would probably be the best thing to ever happen to you in your life and you won't even have a name. I'd open the door and walk out, leaving you to clean yourself up.

A Bad Employee!

It would be just like any other day at the office; you would come in and go to the break room, getting ready for the day, maybe getting some coffee, talking to a couple of your coworkers. You would then go to your desk, start working when I would walk in, asking around about where my husband was, I would walk up to you, asking you if you knew where his office was. You'd get a little nervous, not knowing what to do because you've never talked to somebody so beautiful. You'd stand up, stammering as you suggesting taking me there yourself, I would follow behind you, watching as you fiddled with your glasses, knocking on my husband's door, only to find out he wasn't in. I would roll my eyes, opening the door and inviting you inside with me, you'd ask me why and I would just tell you to come in, and stop being a big baby. I'd close the door behind you, locking it quietly, I would go and sit on the end of my husband's desk, my skirt riding up a little and I would tell you to sit down in one of the chairs in front of me. We would talk for a while. Basically, you are just stammering on about how you love your job and how my husband is amazing, hoping I could get a good word in for you, maybe get you a bonus. I would finally shut you up by standing up and sitting in your lap, rubbing myself against you slightly, asking you if you were gonna spend the whole time talking about my husband when you could be doing something else with me. I would unbutton your shirt slowly, pulling it off of your shoulders, running my hand down your chest slowly. I would start grinding myself against you until your cock got really hard for me, you'd probably be worried that my husband would walk in, but then again that would probably turn you on even more. I would lean down and whisper in your ear how dirty you are, and how mad my husband would be if he found out. I would unzip your pants a little, pulling your cock out, still rubbing myself against it, my underwear moving against your cock. You'd tell me that it felt so good that you liked being dirty, doing it in my husband's office, knowing he could walk in at any second. I would keep kissing on your neck, grinding against you, I would tell you that I wanted you to cum, right here in my husband's chair, leaving a little mess for him to find. I would start bouncing a little, slamming myself against you, making your cock a little sore and you'd grab my hips, pushing me down on you more, and you'd tell me you were really close, and I would keep on pushing myself down against you, and I would tell you to cum, and you would, you would cum all over yourself, and it would get on my panties and on the seat, I would then hop off, going to the door, unlocking it and walking out, telling you to clean yourself up before my husband came back and found you here looking like you jacked off in his office.

Naughty Boy.

I would probably just be out, maybe at the store, just looking for the things that I needed, and I would see you, huddled in some corner, looking like you were messing with yourself and I would come over to you, asking you what the hell you were doing, touching yourself like that in public with people all around. I would drag you by your arm to the nearest family bathroom, pushing you inside and locking the door behind me and looking over at you, telling you that you were gonna get it now because if it was somebody else that saw you, you might be in the back of a cop car for public masturbation. I would push you up against the wall, wrapping my hand around your throat, telling you that I was gonna make you hurt and that you would never get the urge to even scratch yourself in public. I would push my knee up between your thighs, looking you in the eye as I told you to keep quiet because this was gonna hurt. I would then shove my knee up into your crotch, you'd double over, leaning against me and I would push you back up, telling you to suck it up and take it. I would then tighten my hand around your neck, telling you to look at me when I did this, that I wanted to see the pain it caused you. I would keep doing it, watching as you let out groans of pain and then watching as you actually started enjoying it, making me even angrier. I would ask you why you were enjoying it, why you would take advantage of this when you're being punished. I would do it again, and you would just moan so I would stop, leaning back and telling you to take over and start doing this yourself. You'd ask me what I meant, and I would tell you to start pushing yourself down on to my knee. You would then start doing it, really weakly at first but then I would tell you to try it again, this time harder. You would keep doing it, smashing yourself down on me, still enjoying it though. I would pull you closer to me, telling you that you're a very naughty boy for enjoying this, that you're dirty for even being hard because of this. I would keep telling you to go harder, to the point where you were throbbing, your cock would be twitching telling me that you were close. I would then shove my knee up into your balls again, making you lean over and tell me that you were close. I would laugh a little, asking why I cared if you were. I would shove my knee up into your balls again before I backed away, telling you that if you ever thought of doing that kind of thing again, to think of what I did and then I would walk out, leaving you with a throbbing cock waiting to cum.

Birthday Baby Boy

It would probably be the night of your birthday, and we would have spent the day together, going out to someplace nice, just getting out of the house and then finally to end our night we would go to dinner, probably pretty expensive, and we would eat, I'd be sitting across from you, probably reaching my foot across and touching you through your pants, you would start to get hard for me, and u would be able to feel it, I would start digging the heel into your balls, pressing my foot into your cock as we continued to eat, getting you really hard, starting to throb even from how much you wanted me. I would end up stopping so we could finish eating, and after we did we would get in the car, you'd probably be in the driver's seat, I would have my hand on your thigh, rubbing it against you really slowly, squeezing my hand against your thigh and also rubbing it against your hard cock, I would squeeze it really hard, pushing my hand down against your balls, pressing it really hard. We would end up getting home, and I would pull you inside, dragging you back to the bedroom, pushing you down on the bed, I would then undo your tie, using it to tie your hands up. I would then undress, crawling on top of you and rubbing my ass against your cock, grinding myself down against you, you'd probably try and touch me, but you'd soon remember your hands were tied up so I would just keep on rubbing myself against you, smashing my ass against your cock. You would probably start hurting, you'd tell me that it was throbbing really bad and your cock was pressing into your pants, I would probably then pull your pants off along with your boxers, starting rub myself against your cock through my panties, and then I would take them off, shoving them in your mouth and I would then rub myself against you again, pressing myself into you, bouncing up and down on your throbbing cock, my ass smashing against your balls. I would then push my knee up against your balls, leaning down and kissing your neck before I pushed my knee up into you crotch, making you bite down on my panties, trying to let out a groan. I would keep on doing that, smashing my knee into your balls, using my hand to wrap around your cock, pressing my nails into your shaft, jerking you off really hard and fast as I pressed my knee into your balls. You'd try and tell me something, but I would push the panties into your mouth again telling you to be still and quiet. I would keep shoving my knee into your balls, gripping your cock in my hand, jerking you off quickly. I would feel your cock start to throb, and I would start to speed up as I jerked you off, kneeing you even harder. I would probably let you cum just because it was your birthday, finally pressing all of my weight into your balls, jerking you off and letting you cum on your stomach, I would then take my panties out of your mouth, giving you a little kiss on your lips as I untied your hands, laying down next to you and telling you that I might let you fuck me later since I am feeling nice.

It's Lit!

We would be going out for a really nice dinner probably for one of our birthdays or maybe just for a treat, and it would be a fancy one, we would be nice and dressed up, I'd be wearing your favourite dress, and you'd be in some nice pants and a dress shirt. We would get to the restaurant, and we would be waiting for our table, we would be sitting at a bench outside, waiting for our buzzer to go off, letting us know it was our turn to be seated. I would probably be leaning against your shoulder, my hand would be in your lap, rubbing my hand over your thigh slowly, my fingers brushing against your cock, and you'd look at me and ask me what I was doing, and I would just tell you that I'm having fun, being spontaneous. I would keep rubbing you through your pants, squeezing at your cock a little as I did and then the buzzer would go off, and we would have to go inside, or we would lose the table. After we got seated and ordered our drinks, we would probably just be talking about a bunch of random stuff, like we always do, and then I would reach my hand back down again, rubbing you through your pants, leaning in closer so I could kiss on your neck, sucking on it a little to leave some hickeys. I would reach my hand in your pants, wrapping my hand around your cock tightly, starting to jerk you off really slowly, my nails dragging along your shaft. I would keep on doing this, even when the waiter came back around, leaving us our drinks and you'd have to shakily tell him that we needed a little bit more time, trying not to be too obvious at what was happening. I would keep jerking you off really slowly, my nails digging into you as I did. I would then lean my head back, taking my hand off of your cock and patiently waited for the waiter to come back, keeping my hands in my lap. When he came back I would order, taking the lit candle on the table in my hand, rubbing my finger over the class and then I would look over at you, placing your napkin in your lap, pulling your cock out of your pants and then I would blow the candle out, looking into your eyes as I drizzled the hot wax over your cock, you'd probably have to grab the table and bite down a little so you wouldn't groan out, I mean you have to conduct yourself nicely in a high place, and if you didn't, I would make it worse for you. I would then put the candle back on the table, leaving your cock out like that waiting for the hot wax to dry. The waiter would come back with our food, and you'd awkwardly try and cover yourself up, we would eat, and I would completely ignore the fact that your cock was out the entire time. A little bit before we left, I would start scraping the wax off with my nails, leaving it all in the napkin, probably leaving a little bit more of stip to apologize for the mess we left. I would then drag you out to the car, pushing you into the back seat and crawling on top of you, rubbing myself against your cock, pulling it out so I could rub myself against it through my panties, I would start getting wet, and you would be able to feel it through them. I would then move my panties aside, rubbing your tip against my entrance, asking you if you wanted me to fuck you. You would start to beg, telling me you needed my pussy so bad, that you wanted to feel my tight wet pussy around your cock so bad. I would finally end up giving you what you wanted so badly; I would slam myself down against your cock, digging my nails into your chest as I fucked you, grinding my pussy down into your cock, my ass rubbing against your balls. I would keep fucking you, leaning down and kissing along your collar bones, scraping my nails down your chest as I slammed myself against you, and right as I felt you start to pulse inside of me I would get off of you, slamming my knee down against your balls, taking your cock into my hand and squeezing it tightly, jerking you off and it wouldn't take but a few seconds for you to cum right there on your stomach. I might be feeling nice, so I would probably lick it up off of you, and finally, I would drive us home.

The Drunken Joke

Princess Ursula first became aware of an issue that was to greatly shape her life when she was just a young girl of eight.

At the first banquet she was allowed to attend, the hall of her father's castle was alive with festive music and an intoxicating atmosphere of revelry she had previously only ever heard from afar while drifting off to sleep. She was giggling and chattering with the other kids at the children's table and savouring the rich, hearty food when abruptly her father's angry booming voice cut through the general chatter and merriment.

"She'll marry someone better than the son of a knight! Your boy is way below her station, as you ought to know."

Ursula turned and saw her father looking sternly at one of his knights seated next to him. Her father was a large, loud man with a mane of dark hair and beard, lord and master of his domain, and quick to express his displeasure - although Ursula knew that secretly he was really a big sweet softie. An instant hush descended on the hall, and the lute player's fingers stumbled a moment on his strings.

The pink-faced knight bowed as low as he could without putting more of his face than just the tips of his long moustache in his food. "I 'apologise, your 'Eyes! I'm not used to wine. I mushed had too much, to make such a junken droke."

Her father blinked once, then roared in hearty laughter, and slapped the knight on the back. "Sir Oswald has junk to mush wine!" he announced to the hall, his arm now affectionately around the knight's shoulder, "He's making funny drones!"

Everyone had a good laugh at that, including the befuddled Sir Oswald, and the revelry resumed.

Ursula turned back to the other kids. The most fun boy there, Gunter, was Sir Oswald's son. So, ...her father had said no to him marrying her because he wasn't royalty or high nobility. She went quiet and thought about that for a while.

Although she had always assumed she would end up married, she had never given it any thought, and especially not who her husband would actually be. The few times she'd ever imagined a husband, it was only a hazy image of some satisfactory grownup who just pops out of nowhere sometime in her distant future, soon followed by babies. She never imagined that it might be someone she already knew.1

Or that it couldn't be someone she already knew.1

She looked at Gunter. Eyes alight with cheeky mirth, he was telling a story about another time a few years ago when his father had been given wine and ended up getting on his horse backwards. The girls and boys at the table were laughing at the funny bits. She smiled distractedly.

So if she would never marry Gunter, who would she marry? She looked at the other two boys at the table. She thought about all the other boys she had ever met. She didn't particularly want to marry Gunter or anyone else for that matter, but she couldn't think of any boy she liked better. You have to live with your husband, so it's really got to be someone you like, she thought. And of all the boys she knew, he was probably, no; he would have to be the one she liked the best. But she didn't actually know that many boys. She decided this was a matter that needed further thought.

You Gotta Make Your Own Fairytale

Ursula had a lovely nanny named Gertrude, who had been teaching and looking after her for as long as she could remember, and who told the best bedtime stories. Some she read, some she told from memory, and she made some up too.

Many of the stories were fairytales about a girl, who may or may not be a princess, and in the end, she would always marry a prince — even if he might sometimes start out like a beast or frog. Many of these girls somehow managed to really irritate a witch, who would try to murder her, or at least imprison her somehow. In a couple of stories the witch trapped the princess in a deep sleep she couldn't wake from, and in several others in a tower without a door, only accessible by flying broomstick.... or in one case by ridiculously long hair. The tower often had extra security too, such as a dragon to guard it, or a magical wall of thorns. But no matter how far away the prison and how well defended, a prince would without fail always show up to rescue and then promptly marry the girl.

Ursula understood these were just stories and real-life was different. She didn't expect she would ever offend a witch, and nor did she go around kissing frogs. Nevertheless, these stories were still an influence on her several years later when her father decided she was of marriageable age and started recruiting eligible suitors.

The realm of Lundgren where she lived wasn't a kingdom but only a small principality, ruled by her father the prince. It was part of a group of several other small principalities and duchies united under a defence pact. Under the agreement, none of the princes or dukes could be known as a king, even though each was the absolute ruler of their realm. In Lundgren, like in several others, there were no nobles of rank higher than a knight, apart from the royal family. And since Ursula's father had shown on the night of Sir Oswald's "junk droke" that he would not permit her to marry a knight, she knew her husband would be from another realm, and she would go to live with him there far from home.

Her father sent messages out to all the royal courts and noble castles of Europe to invite suitors for Ursula. Replies started coming back. The answer was always no. Sometimes the family didn't have an unbetrothed son the right age, but sometimes even though they did, they were not interested in having him pursue Ursula.

At first, she was a bit relieved, but after the "no"s started piling up, it finally got to her. One evening she asked her father, "Why are they not interested in me when they haven't even met me?"

"My darling girl, it's not you they're not interested in, it's Lundgren. My messengers have been describing you as fair of face and form, pure and kind of heart, with beautiful bright blue eyes framed by lustrous dark hair. I composed that myself. Do you like it? It's just the truth. But there's not much great to be said about Lundgren, I'm afraid."

"What do you mean? What's wrong with Lundgren? Why would they judge me for being Lundgrenian?"

"Power and money," he answered. "Lundgren is small and unimportant. You've seen us on a map — we're tiny. Royal and noble families try to marry their children into the most powerful families they can. Surely you know that, right?"

She thought about this a moment, and then asked, "Is that why you said I could never marry Sir Oswald's son?"

"That still makes me laugh!" her father chuckled. "It wasn't just what he said — you should've seen the look on his face!" He chuckled a bit more. "Anyway, yes, you're right."

"But why do they care how powerful the family is?" she asked.

"To get powerful allies of course," he answered. "If a realm is weak and isolated, one of its neighbours might invade. It's like

114

our defence pact. Together we're stronger. Families want to ally with powerful families, so no one would dare attack them."

She thought again for a moment, then asked, "But why does anyone attack anyone in the first place? If no one ever attacked, then everyone would be safe."

"Oh, I agree! But to answer your question: some who start wars are just as evil as the witches in those stories Gertrude used to tell you, and don't care who they hurt if they can make themselves more important. But life's complicated. Others who start wars actually aren't that bad. They conquer and make their realm more powerful only to better protect it against attack by others."

After a moment, Ursula asked, "Does that mean no one's going to want to marry me?"

"We're still waiting on replies. I'm sure we'll get someone."

Again she thought for a moment.

"What if we finally get just one eligible suitor, but I really don't like him? What then?"

"I wouldn't like that. I would hope to choose the best marriage possible. But in this example you give, there is simply no one better available. So you would have to marry that one, I think. Actually, it would depend on what I think of the man."

She took a moment to think.

"But if there were several suitors that you were happy with, what then? If there were say a dozen princes or dukes paying suit, and all of them were acceptable to you, would you let me choose then?"

"Dozens? Ha! Yes, I would."

"Ok, I know what to do," she said, and ran away, leaving her father in mystified amusement.

The room next to hers was Gertrude's. She pounded on the door.

"Is that you, my little turnip?"

"Yeah, can I come in?"

"Of course."

Ursula had the door open and shut again behind her in an instant.

"Goodness, what's the matter?" asked Gertrude, sitting on the edge of her bed with a book in hand, motherly concern showing on her kindly face.

"Gerty, I'm worse than a turnip, I'm a princess without a suitor!"

"Well maybe I'm selfish, but I can't help it — I want you to stay here with me a bit longer, so I'm in no hurry to get you married off," she replied.

"I'm not in a hurry! I just want someone I like. So I want you to kidnap me!"

"Err... what do you mean?"

"I want you to imprison me in a tower!"

"Heavens! Whatever for?!"

"To make all the princes come to rescue me!"

"Oh! I see. But we don't have a tower."

"We do! I'll get Daddy to repair the old ruined one on the hill near the lake! I mean, if he says yes."

"Well, but... ok, I guess... but what do you actually want me to do?"

"Pretend you're the witch who's keeping me locked up! Here's the plan:

Kidnapped by a Wicked Witch

After Ursula had explained the plan to Gertrude and her father, and convinced him to give it a try, it only took about a month to repair and clean out the old tower. Then it was time to stage the kidnapping. They wanted lots of witnesses so the story would spread far and wide. So her father invited all his knights and several of the neighbouring rulers and their families to a huge banquet. By the time of the banquet, they had everything ready.

It was a grand affair, with great entertainment from minstrels and bards, jesters and acrobats. There was loads of delicious mutton cooked in honey and pepper and vinegar, fried pastries full of salty ginger pork and crushed almonds, boiled eggs with mustard, roast pheasant with fresh bread and butter, and plenty of beer and wine.

When her father gave the signal, by loudly asking, "Another glass of wine, Sir Oswald?", a few servants put out most of the torches on the wall, so the hall became quite dark. Under the distraction of the mirth that erupted following this question, with calls of "Hasn't he had to mush already?!" and "When will you tell us a junk droke?!", the darkness was barely noticed. Nor did anyone notice Ursula move into position against the wall and a rope slide down to her. She fastened it to a harness hidden under her clothes, then gave a little tug to signal she was ready. Up above her was a large window with the shutters open, letting the smoke out and the summer evening breeze in.

Suddenly there was a loud bang and a flash from the window and a cloud of smoke, followed by shocked silence, broken by an evil cackling laugh. As the smoke cleared, they saw a cloaked figure with a long nose and chin in a pointy hat sitting on a broom.

"It's a witch!"

"Witch!!"

"It's a witch!"

"Prince Hendrick!" she cried. "I'm here to take my revenge on you! Say goodbye to your only daughter! I will keep her locked in the tower near the lake! Hee, he hee!!!"

Princess Ursula screamed and struggled as she was lifted by the rope up to the witch at the window. There were another flash and bang and a cloud of smoke, and when it cleared, there was nothing there to be seen but the stars in the night sky.

"After them!" bellowed the prince.

Servants and knights and others rushed out of the hall and through a doorway that leads to a balcony running under the window, but Ursula and the witch were nowhere to be seen.

"Great job, Gerty!" Ursula thanked her nanny. "You even scared me a bit!"

They were hiding in a secret room behind a large tapestry hanging on the wall near the entranceway to the balcony. Running from this room was a secret tunnel that leads all the way to the tower. Gertrude took off the pointy hat, removed her fake chin and nose and dropped them inside it, and tucked the hat and the broom under her arm. "Right," she said, "Let's go and lock you in the tower!"

Word of the kidnapping spread like wildfire. It became the talk of Europe. Castles everywhere started taking security precautions against the abduction of their daughters by witches. Everyone was saying that some brave prince really ought to rescue Ursula, and young men bragged to each other how they would go about defeating the witch. Her father sent letters asking for help and offering her hand in marriage to anyone courageous enough to rescue her — provided he was of rank higher than a knight.

And this time princes and other nobles started showing up at the tower.

My Kidnap Brings all the Boys to the Tower

The first to arrive was Duke Fredrik, eldest son of the Duke of Blatzenkolt, riding on an enormous white charger, his armour shining in the sun, his shield painted white with a blue unicorn. Behind him on a horse packed with camp gear and extra weapons rode his young squire.

Ursula and Gertrude peeked out through the narrow slit windows when they heard the horses' hooves on the rocky approach to the tower. "Yes!" said Ursula. "That didn't take too long! — this is going to work Gerty!"

"The little squire looks terrified, poor fellow," said Gertrude. "I feel a bit guilty."

The lad was fearfully scanning the sky for incoming witches. His face had gone so pale it almost made his flaxen blond hair look dark.

The pair halted a distance from the tower, which was situated at the top of a rocky pinnacle because the climb was now too steep.

"Keep your wits about you, Lukas," they heard Duke Fredrik say, "remember there may be a dragon."

Lukas was already looking around nervously, his hand on the hilt of his sword.

"And I would love nothing more than to slay it!" added Duke Fredrik enthusiastically.

He looked up at the tower, then at the rocky climb to reach it.

"You stay here with the horses," he ordered and started climbing.

"He's coming!" said Ursula.

"He looks a bit like you," said Gertrude, "if you were a strapping dashing young man."

When he reached the bottom of the tower, they went out onto the balcony that encircled the room at the top and knelt to peek down through the peepholes in the floor. They watched, moving from peephole to peephole, as Duke Fredrik did one lap around the base of the tower.

"Well, there's no door to knock on," he called to the squire.

He looked up and shouted, "Witch! I am here to free Princess Ursula. I demand you release her to me unharmed!"

"Yeah, right! As if!!" yelled back Gertrude in a witchy voice, "What do you think this is?! You have to rescue her, you big ninny!"

"Gerty!" hissed Ursula, that might be my future husband, you're insulting!"

"This is too much fun!" she giggled.

"Foul witch!" shouted Duke Fredrik as his squire crossed himself and drew his sword. "I give you this one last chance to surrender, or have your ugly head cut off!"

He drew his sword and held it aloft, so it caught the sun.

"Very impressive!" whispered Gertrude.

"He is quite the questing hero, isn't he?" giggled Ursula.

"How do you think you're going to do that all the way from down there?" asked witchy Gertrude.

Duke Fredrik was silent a moment. "I don't know," he admitted. "But I have you surrounded."

"Aren't you forgetting my broomstick?"

He thought a moment, then called back, "I challenge you to transform into a dragon and come down to do battle, so that I may slay you!"

"I'd rather just stay up here, thanks," she replied.

"Have you no honour?" he asked desperately.

"Well... only just a bit, I suppose. Enough to get by, but, yeah, not that much."

"Gerty, you're making fun of him!" scolded Ursula.

"I can't help it! It's too much fun!"

Duke Fredrik stood there awhile.

"Witch, this will be your undoing!" he finally declared.

Gertrude didn't answer.

After a minute, Duke Fredrik asked, "Will you not please just fight me?"

"Nup! Not happening!" replied Gertrude.

"Then you are a coward!"

"Maybe. Anyway, I'm not coming down."

Finally, the exasperated Fredrik shouted, "Damn you, witch!" and climbed back down to his squire.

"She won't fight! Can you believe it?!"

"How dishonourable!" said a very relieved Lukas.

"We shall have to build a ladder," announced Duke Fredrik. "Get out the axe and the ropes."

"Gerty, we can't let him climb up now! If he does, I'll have to marry him. I won't get to choose my husband. You've got to stop him!"

"How can I stop him building a ladder? I'm not really a witch, remember!"

"No, you've got to push it back down every time they put it up. I can't do it! I'm supposed to want to be rescued!"

The next day, as Duke Fredrik and his squire worked on their ladder, the Prince of Greznig showed up on his own white horse and in his own shining armour, accompanied by several mounted men-at-arms.

Hearing the clatter on the stones, Ursula and Gertrude rushed to the narrow windows to watch.

His shield bore his coat of arms, the left half red, the right half blue, and a golden lion on each. The fluttering banner held aloft by one of his men was the same, as was his cloak.

"Wow!" said Gertrude, "I bet this one's a prince!"

Duke Fredrik and Lukas had stopped work on their ladder and were standing watching the prince approach.

The horses pulled up in front of them.

"Greetings, Your Highness," said Duke Fredrik and bowed.

"Greetings ..... Duke...? Lord....?"

"Duke Fredrik, eldest son of the Duke of Blatzenkolt."

"Greetings Duke," said the prince. "As you seem to know, I am Gerhard, Prince of Greznig. I assume you are here to rescue the princess too?"

"Yes, I am. And I got here first!"

Prince Gerhard looked at the still very unfinished ladder, giving his sparse brown beard a few absent-minded strokes. Duke Frederick's own beard would have been about as sparse, but he thought it looked foolish like that, so he was cleanly shaven.

"But you haven't rescued her. Have you ever seen the witch?"

"She spoke to me. She refuses to fight, the coward!"

"Repugnant things they are, witches," said the prince. "Men! Start building me a ladder!"

They jumped to action.

"Hey, that's not fair!" objected Duke Fredrik.

"There's a princess that needs rescuing!" replied Prince Gerhard. "The race is on!!"

"They have a ladder building race!" said Ursula.

"This might get tricky," said Gertrude, imagining two ladders to push off.

Prince Gerhard turned and headed towards the tower.

"Gerty, behave yourself this time!" said Ursula.

"Witch! I demand the release of Princess Ursula. My men are building a ladder even as I speak. But if you release the princess to me now, we will not harm you."

"Harm me?! You'll be turned into frogs!"

"I don't believe you! Why don't you demonstrate on Duke Fredrik over there?"

"Ha! Very crafty!" cackled Gertrude. "I'll demonstrate on anyone fool enough to climb up here."

Prince Gerhard turned and went back to his men. He ordered one to go and buy saws, timber axes, hammers, and lots of nails. The others continued cutting down trees with their firewood hatchets.

The next day Herman, eldest son of the Baron of Tilsdorf, turned up, then within a few minutes so did Prince Hertel of Holstein.

After they each made their own unsuccessful demands for Ursula's release, Prince Hertel suggested to the others, "Why don't we all join forces? Together we're stronger."

"No," replied Prince Gerhard. "We can't all marry her. So we can't all rescue her."

"I'll share the glory of this heroic deed with no man!" proclaimed Duke Fredrik. "I only wish there were a dragon as well, that I might slay it too."

In the end, the newcomers joined the ladder building race.

And by the end of the day, so too had Prince Andreas of Kurnst, Prince Konrad of Litznich, and Count Kristoff of Basselfelt.

That made four princes, the son of a duke, one count and the son of a baron still in contention. Ursula couldn't believe how well her plan was working.

Lightning Source UK Ltd.
Milton Keynes UK
UKHW021252261120
374146UK00015B/1275